Community Psychology
and Mental Health

Contributors

Daniel Adelson, Associate Professor of Psychology in Residence, University of California, San Francisco; Research Associate, Institute of Human Development, University of California, Berkeley

Lenin A. Baler, Head, Community Mental Health Unit; Associate Professor of Community Mental Health, University of Michigan School of Public Health

Timothy W. Costello, Deputy Mayor-City Administrator, City of New York; on leave Professor of Management and Psychology, Graduate School of Business Administration, New York University

John B. Enright, Assistant Clinical Professor of Medical Psychology, Department of Psychiatry, University of California, San Francisco

J. Douglas Grant, New Careers Development Organization, Oakland, California

Joan Grant, New Careers Development Organization, Oakland, California

Leonard Hassol, Professor of Community Psychology, Wheaton College

Betty L. Kalis, Senior Psychologist, Langley Porter Neuropsychiatric Institute, California Department of Mental Hygiene; Associate Clinical Professor of Medical Psychology, Department of Psychiatry, University of California, San Francisco

James G. Kelly, Professor of Psychology and Research Associate, Institute for Social Research, University of Michigan

Donald C. Klein, Program Director, Center for Community Affairs, National Training Laboratories, Washington, D.C.

Lester M. Libo, Associate Professor and Director, Behavioral Science Program, Department of Psychiatry, University of New Mexico School of Medicine

Herbert Lipton, Associate Professor of Psychology and Faculty Coordinator, Community Psychology Training Program, Boston University

Howard E. Mitchell, Director, Human Resources Program, University of Pennsylvania; 1907 Foundation Professor in Urbanism and Human Resources

J. R. Newbrough, Associate Professor and Director, Community Psychology Program, George Peabody College for Teachers

William C. Rhodes, Professor of Psychology, University of Michigan

Nevitt Sanford, Scientific Director, Wright Institute, Berkeley, California

Theodore R. Sarbin, Professor of Psychology, University of California, Santa Cruz

Julius Seeman, Professor of Psychology, George Peabody College for Teachers

Charles D. Spielberger, Professor of Psychology and Director, Doctoral Program in Clinical Psychology, Florida State University

Robert F. Stepbach, Jr., Clinical and Consulting Psychologist, Nashville, Tennessee

Sheldon S. Zalkind, Professor of Psychology, Baruch College, City University of New York

Community Psychology and Mental Health

PERSPECTIVES AND CHALLENGES

Edited by

Daniel Adelson and Betty L. Kalis
UNIVERSITY OF CALIFORNIA, SAN FRANCISCO

CHANDLER PUBLISHING COMPANY
An Intext Publisher • Scranton, Pennsylvania 18515

117800

Copyright © 1970 by Chandler Publishing Company

Pages 177-207 are copyright by Timothy W. Costello and Sheldon S. Zalkind.

All Rights Reserved

International Standard Book Number 0-8102-0002-3 (Hard Cover)

International Standard Book Number 0-8102-0377-4 (Soft Cover)

Library of Congress Catalog Card No. 70-90275

Printed in the United States of America

COVER DESIGN BY R. Keith Richardson

Contents

Preface

About five years have passed since a group of thirty-nine psychologists, meeting at Swampscott, Massachusetts, to discuss education for psychologists in community mental health, struck forth in new directions and created a new subarea of psychology—community psychology.

Whatever there is in a name, somehow the idea of "community psychology" seemed to those at the conference to provide the key concept for responding to crises in the community, to stirrings within psychology itself, and most particularly to what has been called the third revolution in mental health. And it is significant that the conference conceived community mental health to be only one of the subspecialties of community psychology—this by a group of psychologists whose primary interests were in the mental-health field.

In this volume we are concerned with mental health, but our emphasis is on the perspectives and challenges to mental health which community psychology presents. If community psychology in some of its central aspects is a response to developments in mental health, it also goes beyond mental health, as indeed, "community mental health" may be said to be different from "community psychiatry." The study (*ology*) of the mind in the community is different from the treatment (*iatry*) of the mind in the community. This seemingly small difference is of prime significance for orientation, for theory, for research, and for practice.

This collection, which began with most of the papers from two symposia on community psychology at the 1966 meetings of the American Psychological Association, grew to include other papers especially prepared for this book and previously published papers, as we tried to make the book representative of current theory, practice, research, and teaching in this rapidly burgeoning field.

The contributors to this volume come to community psychology from many vantage points and from varied settings. Yet some central orientations and approaches do emerge which are of significance not only for mental health but for psychology as it develops new pathways in relation to the multifaceted conditions and problems of the community.

Daniel Adelson
Betty L. Kalis

Community Psychology
and Mental Health

The Emergence of Community Psychology: A Question of Models

This is a time of crisis, of change and demands for change in the larger community, on university and college campuses, and in those professions which have been most directly involved in working with social and human problems. The emergence of "community psychology" as a subspecialty of psychology may be seen as a major response to this current crisis.

Community psychology may also be seen as the culmination of deep-rooted developments in psychology and in the social sciences, whether we date the beginnings of these developments from Kurt Lewin's call for action research in the 1930's, John Dewey's concern with "Psychology and Social Practice" (the title of his 1899 presidential address to the American Psychological Association), or farther back than that in terms of the development of the democratic idea and advances in science.

This collection stems initially from two symposia on community psychology at the meetings of the American Psychological Association in 1966.[1] The book reflects some perspectives on the concerns and approaches of this new area of psychology—broadly in the field of mental health and more specifically with respect to (1) historical evolution and philosophy, (2) theoretical points of view, (3) research and action on community and social problems, and (4)

---

[1]Chapters 2, 3, 4, 15, 16, and 17 in this book were presented at one or the other of the symposia, "Issues and Trends in Community Psychology" and "Community Psychology: How Much Commitment," 74th Annual Convention of the American Psychological Association, New York City, September 2-3, 1966. Chapters 5, 9, 10, 12, 13, and 14 are original publications in this book. With the exception of Chapters 8, 11, 17, and 18, the chapters have been revised and edited for publication.

1

issues and trends in education and training. These four areas form the four major parts into which this book is divided.

The perspectives offered here are not necessarily limited to matters of mental health or community mental health. Nonetheless, the title does give the reader a notion of the major focus of this volume and serves to remind us that what might be called the official birth of community psychology took place at the Boston Conference on the Education of Psychologists for Community Mental Health.[2]

While these are varied perspectives, a number of key issues and concerns are repeatedly raised which merit mention here.

A central issue with which contributors to this volume are concerned is the fundamental orientation to human and social problems of this subarea of psychology. Shall it be "pathology" oriented, or shall it be "growth" oriented? Adelson raises this question in contrasting a "traditional treatment" with a "growth and development" model. In emphasizing the shift from man's adapting himself to the existing social world to man's modifying social reality in order to accomodate a greater range of social needs, Rhodes points up the implications of such a growth orientation for practice. Kalis's development of crisis theory emphasizes a growth model as well.

With the emphasis on growth comes a shift to theories, concepts, and constructs concerned with "man in his environment." Virtually all the chapters in the book demonstrate this focus on ecological theory or on the individual in society. This is particularly illustrated by Kelly's development of ecological theory, by Sarbin's role-theory approach, and by Adelson's chapter on self-valuation, social valuation, and self-identity.

The viewpoint provided by psychodynamic theory remains nonetheless a fundamental base and may be one of the special contributions of the psychologist to the understanding and solution of community problems. Sanford's chapter on alcoholism demonstrates the psychodynamic orientation, as does Kalis's paper on crisis theory, though this latter theory also has its ecological orientation, and Sanford draws clearly the implications of his approach for change in the legal and educational systems of the community.

[2]C. C. Bennett, Lurleen S. Anderson, S. Cooper, L. Hassol, D. C. Klein, & G. Rosenblum. *Community psychology: a report of the Boston conference on the education of psychologists for community mental health*, May, 1965. Boston: Boston Univer. Press, 1966.

The growth model is also bringing to the fore new techniques and new approaches for psychologists who work in the community and its subsystems. Examples in this book are the multiple functions described by Libo, the sensitivity-group approach used by Hassol in bridging the gap between adults and adolescents, the multiproblem neighborhood project proposed by Rhodes and his colleagues, the research as participation model of the Grants, and the model which appears to raise most questions with respect to the traditional stance of clinical psychology—the self-help group as discussed by Enright.

Concomitant with the emphasis on growth, the ecological orientation, and the new techniques is a move toward research and action on problems of prevention via education and on urban and neighborhood problems and the larger populations at risk as described by Mitchell of Philadelphia, Costello and Zalkind of New York, and Rhodes, Seeman, Spielberger, and Stepbach in their chapter on the multiproblem neighborhood.

These changing emphases have implications for approaches to and problems in training and the setting in which training takes place. Kalis emphasizes this in her description and discussion of the Langley Porter program. Lipton and Klein also discuss and clarify problems with respect to training in describing students from the clinical areas as contrasted with the social-psychological and personality areas.

What kind of preparation will this new type of psychologist need? What will be his professional identity? To what extent is he an action researcher? a participant-conceptualizer? or, broadly, a change agent—combining all these aspects? Newbrough raises this issue of future emphasis in community psychology: Will it be research or practice? And Baler, in discussing research, relates this question to the problem of the relationship between theory and practice.

With respect to training, the question of the psychologist's unique contribution and identity, in the light of the multidisciplinary base of community work (in law, sociology, anthropology, and social-work techniques), comes to the fore. This issue is related to the trend toward interdisciplinary training. Many programs now provide community mental-health training on an interdisciplinary basis to nurses, psychologists, psychiatrists, and social workers.

Mitchell's experience in Philadelphia where psychologists, unlike members of other disciplines, failed to respond to a call for work on urban problems also raises this question of the self-image and self-identity of psychologists in general and of the community psychologist in particular.

This volume is also offered as a contribution to university-community integration. The community is looking to the university for help in understanding and solving a variety of social and community crises and problems, and the university is seeking ways not only of doing research but also of taking action with respect to these problems. A number of the chapters suggest and describe how, to use Mitchell's phrase, the university can be a principal agent of democracy in the community.

In this regard, it may be noted that community psychology is concerned with broader problems than those encompassed by the phrase "community mental health." Varied as are the points of view contained here, they represent only a limited segment of community-psychology interests.

Finally, while this book offers perspectives on community psychology, the field of community mental health includes many other professions as practitioners, researchers, and teachers. It is hoped that this volume will have meaning for these other disciplines as well as for psychology.

I

EVOLUTION
AND PHILOSOPHICAL
ROOTS OF COMMUNITY
PSYCHOLOGY

Community psychology, its evolution and viewpoints, is developed in several ways in this first part: (1) historically, (2) in relation to change and flux on the current scene, (3) as a subspecialty of psychology, and (4) in a semiautobiographical account of one individual's development into a community psychologist.

In Chapter 1, Adelson provides a community-psychology viewpoint of a concept of comprehensive community mental health, tracing its philosophical-historical origins in the evolution of the democratic idea, in scientific advances, and in man's increasing understanding of the nature of man. He then proposes a growth-and-development model for practice and research in community mental health, differentiating its emphases from those of the more traditional medical-treatment model. This contrast suggests a number of approaches and raises a number of issues to which many of the succeeding chapters return.

Rhodes's chapter reviews developments on the current scene. It discusses the problems of professional guild commitment as these relate to human problems which have no guild boundaries, the question of the fit between the individual and his social world, and the shifting concern to modifying social reality. Chapter 2 also describes the emerging role of the university with respect to the community—a theme taken up again in this part by Mitchell.

From these broader historical and contemporary contexts the next two chapters focus more specifically on community psychology as a new subspecialty of psychology and on the evolution of one man into a community psychologist.

Newbrough, in Chapter 3, traces the origins of community psychology as a subspecialty of psychology deriving from applied psychology. He uses

Bucher and Strauss's process model for the analysis of the development of professions to describe the character of specialization in this particular field. The issue of the primary work of community psychology (whether it is to be service or research) and the question of the validity of traditional techniques for providing service are raised. The development of counseling psychology as a paradigm of what community psychologists will need to concern themselves with is cited. In acknowledging the growing ecological emphasis of the field, the chapter refers to the idiographic versus nomothetic considerations which have hampered sociological ecologists. Newbrough is also concerned with primary training needs and with the research methods to be used in the practice of community psychology.

In the concluding chapter of this part, Chapter 4, Mitchell provides a personalized account of his development into a community psychologist from an initially clinical base. He emphasizes the need for psychologists to be more directly involved at various levels of decision making and in planning service and research. Noting the two-way interaction of the university and the community, he suggests that the school or college can become the principal agency of democracy in the community. The very title of his program, "human resources," suggests the broad range of community-psychology concerns, and may be seen as going beyond the bounds of community mental health. Mitchell's contribution also raises fundamental issues for the preparation of psychologists. Psychological personnel failed to respond when contacted for a pilot project for the Urban Job Corps Training Centers, whereas students in other fields were eager to be part of this program. What role models is psychology providing for attracting those students who wish to be involved in action as well as research in the community? Mitchell's career and activities provide one significant example of such a role model.

CHAPTER 1

A Concept of Comprehensive Community Mental Health

Daniel Adelson

I have been asked in this talk to and with you today to speak on a concept of comprehensive community mental health and also, in particular, on an underlying philosophy for such a concept. I have searched over the weeks for a philosophy to share with you, and ever and again I return to the great concerns of mankind—to problems of freedom, of brotherhood, and of equality. In a culturally pluralistic society, it may be considered of some significance that this important workshop coincides with one of the most sacred holidays in the Judeo-Christian tradition, Passover. Passover, as you know, is the celebration of a people's casting off the bonds of slavery, of their struggle over forty long years in the desert to reach their own land, of their self-liberation, of their search for a community and an identity of their own as a free and autonomous people. It is essentially, then, a holiday marking man's historical quest for freedom. But not a freedom without bounds—for even as the group led by Moses were in process of removing themselves from slavery and moving toward freedom, they were handed from Sinai the two tablets containing the Ten Commandments. The freedom celebrated at Passover is a freedom under law. In a democratic society, as contrasted with an anarchic or authoritarian society, there can be no other way than freedom under the rule of law.

Ernest Jones (1955, p. 364) has vividly described Freud's iden-

Keynote paper presented at the Work Conference in Graduate Education in Psychiatric-Mental Health Nursing, University of Maryland, Baltimore, April 24, 1967.

tification with Moses and in particular Freud's interpretation of
the statue of Moses by Michelangelo as "not intended to represent
Moses as about to start up and punish the disobedient people"
(who were dancing around their golden calf) but, contrary to the
version in the Bible, as struggling successfully against an inward
passion for the sake of preserving the precious tablets which he
had observed were about to slip from his grasp. Here, indeed, is
a symbolization of commitment to the rule of law as essential to
freedom.[1]

FREEDOM UNDER THE RULE OF LAW

The evolution of a community's laws over time is one of the
major threads through which the community builds its sense of
common destiny. As Louisa Howe has pointed out:

Respectful regard for the past lends added symbolic significance to the
charter, constitution or contract by which the community (be it a family,
a city, a profession, an organization, or a nation) was first established and
by which its destiny continues to be shaped. The community remains
bound by this charter, necessary changes being made through successive
reinterpretations and occasional revisions of the original document. These
semi-sacred writings provide an essential touchstone for testing the acceptability of new provisions or practices. The viability of the community's charter, together with an accumulating body of laws or rules and
customary procedures, likewise contributes to the members' sense of the
continuity between past and present, to their confidence in facing the
future, and to their feeling of kinship with other members of the community, whether the living, the dead, or those yet to be born.
It is of great importance also to note that in human communities it is
the law which defines who the community's members shall be, where the
lines are that mark the community's boundaries, and under what conditions the rights of membership (the rights of a citizen, for example) can
be gained—or lost. The law prescribes certain obligations in return for the
rights of membership that it bestows, and it is only to those who are
judged capable of fulfilling their obligations that the prospect of common
destiny is held forth (Howe, 1964, p. 21).

Howe points out further that crises of various sorts may serve
either to heighten or to lessen the sense of community. During
crises, change designed to prevent the recurrence of similar catas-
trophic events may be instituted; but it is also possible that sacrifi-

---

[1]The concept of freedom under the rule of law should not be confused with the
cry for law and order which may indicate a disregard for the essential freedoms
outlined in the Bill of Rights, other amendments to the Constitution, and elsewhere
in the body of law.

cial scapegoats may be found, and there is danger that

[Leaders with an authoritarian bent may] make use of this increased fluidity of community structure to substitute their own decrees for the previously established judicial and law-making procedures. Although certain formal semblances of the latter may still be retained, these mainly serve to mock, rather than to safeguard, the principles of justice and equality. In the absence of respect for these principles the community is weakened, with increasing mistrust taking the place of the earlier feeling of elation aroused by common pursuit of a high mission (Howe, 1964, p. 22).

One of the major foundations of community, then, as well as of community mental health is in the evolving law, the changing views of what the law should be, and what "freedom under the rule of law" means. This, indeed, would seem at first glance to be a paradox—that freedom is only freedom within bounds—but it is a paradox which has been resolved over time through two major historical movements which also form the deeper roots of a philosophy and concept of comprehensive community mental health: the growth and development of the democratic idea, and the growth of science and man's constantly increasing understanding of the nature of man and of the social, psychological, and biological factors which may hinder or promote man's relations with himself and with his fellow man. We sort out these major streams, while recognizing fully that they form one gestalt. Ultimately, both scientific and democratic advancement rest on a faith in man, in his rational processes, and "in his capacity when in an environment which permits him freedom of speech, communication, and inquiry, to grow in his understanding of the physical world and of the world of relations between man and man" (Adelson, 1964b, p. 454).

THE SPIRIT OF FREE INQUIRY

Under the impact of scientific inquiry, man has broadened his views of his relations to the natural world, has changed his religious beliefs and practices, his political systems and economic arrangements, and, in our time, has increasingly deepened his understanding of the psychological, social, and biological factors which influence both his intrapsychic and his interpersonal relations. These changing views have been characterized by a movement from dogma to dependence on rational processes, a movement from authority in a hierarchical world based on inherited and conferred status to authority based on achieved status and merit,[2] a movement from relatively closed, undifferentiated, monolithic societies to societies characterized by pluralism, openness, and growth. Increasingly, we have insight into the conditions under which it is possible or not possible to "love thy neighbor as thyself" and into the obstacles which stand in the way of building the "many mansions" which are a possibility in "my Father's house."

Let us briefly sketch a few of the highlights of this movement. In Western civilization, it may be said to have begun with the impulse given to free inquiry in the city-states of Greece, particularly by its great philosophers: Socrates, who enjoined us "Know thyself"; Plato, whose *Republic* provided us with our first major projection of a sane community or society; and Aristotle, who was our first great empirical scientist. In the Greek city-states we find concern also with those aspects of democracy which continue to need thinking and resolution today: the question of direct and indirect representation; the question of who did and who did not belong to the democratic community (those who did not were labeled "barbarians"); and the question of freedom of dialogue and inquiry.

Copernicus (1473-1543) may be said to have taken the first great step toward modern science—a science based on observation, experimentation, and measurement. The Copernican revolution dealt a blow to the view of the earth and its heavens as central to the universe. Man and the world he had built around him were decentralized; but in losing the hierarchy of the heavens, man gained greater faith in his own rational powers.

As the spirit of free inquiry was applied to church and religion in the sixteenth and seventeenth centuries, there was a transfer of authority from the church to the Bible, with individual right of interpretation—a right considerably strengthened by the invention of the printing press in 1452.

These changes, indeed, eventually resulted in new architectural arrangements, which bolstered man's more egalitarian relationship with minister and fellow man:

the dimly-lit, vast auditorium of a Gothic Catholic cathedral, bathed in colors and symbols, faces a bright candle-lit stage and its richly costumed

[2]See Gardner (1962, pp. 3-10); see also Thompson (1953).

celebrant; this is the necessary background for the mysterious sacrament of the mass for the newly growing medieval town and its representative actor. But the daylit, small and unadorned meeting hall of the Congregationalist, facing its central pulpit, fits the belief that the chief mystery is preaching the Word to a group that religiously governs itself. And the little square seating arrangement of the Quakers confronting one another is an environment where it is hoped that, when people are gathered in meditation, the Spirit itself will descend anew. In this sequence of three plans, there is a whole history of dogma and society (Goodman & Goodman, 1960, pp. 3-4).

Similarly, as the spirit of inquiry was applied to governmental and political forms, absolute monarchy gave way to the idea of representative government in the eighteenth and nineteenth centuries. In all these areas, the movement was toward the abolition of privilege and the rise of constitutional liberty, and away from authority based on status toward an authority based on reason and merit.

Beginning in the nineteenth century also, under the impact of the urbanization and industrialization which stemmed from scientific inquiry, the movement from country to city, from community to mass society, we find the spirit of scientific inquiry turning to concern with man's relations to his group and community. We find the beginnings of sociology as a separate science early in the century, and of psychology as a separate science toward the end of the century. And here we begin to find the more immediate predecessors of the current revolution in community psychiatry and community mental health.

We are less than two hundred years from the Paris which nurtured Pinel's humanitarian views—views which led him to strike off the chains of the insane at the Bicêtre in 1793. "The mentally sick," he said, "far from being guilty people deserving of punishment, are sick people whose miserable state deserves all the consideration that is due to suffering humanity. One should try with the most simple methods to restore their reason" (quoted in R. W. White, 1948, p. 9).

One hundred years have gone by since the 1867 English Poor Law was passed—a law which the founder of modern nursing, Florence Nightingale, had worked hard to effect. After the bill was passed, she wrote to the Reverend Mother Bermondrey:

We have obtained some things, the removal of 2,000 lunatics, 80 fever and smallpox cases and all the remaining children out of the workhouses—

(and the providing for them out of a common fund in order to relieve the rates), the paying of all salaries of Medical Officers, Matrons, Nurses, etc., out of a Metropolitan (not parochial) rate ... Also—the removing all other sick into separate buildings which are to be improved—and constituting fresh boards of guardians for these sick with nominees from the Poor Law Board. This is a beginning ... (Frank, 1953, p. 229).

The same year, 1867, was also the year of publication of Marx's *Das Kapital,* a book which has so profoundly affected the thinking and action of major portions of our world.

We are only three score and ten years away from 1897, the year that Freud began the self-analysis in Vienna that provided man with a way of unraveling the inner skeins of the psyche which, indeed, were often tighter and stronger than the outer chains which Pinel had removed. In that same year, Durkheim in France published *Suicide,* the first social-scientific investigation of the factors related to a major form of social pathology, an investigation of prime theoretical import even today. Two years later, in 1899, John Dewey, the great philosopher of democracy, entitled his address as president of the American Psychological Association "Psychology and Social Practice," a title which was a harbinger of the flowering in the 1900's up to our own time of the sciences and practices concerned with psychosocial man.

For Dewey, as for William James and George Mead, two other pragmatist philosophers, the concept of *self* was central—self as social in origin, self as active, dynamic, reconstructing, and reorganizing, and self-realization as in Dewey's *Democratic Education* (Dewey, 1916; as interpreted by Thompson, 1953). Mead observed:

It is often assumed that democracy is an order of society in which those personalities which are sharply differentiated will be eliminated, that everything will be ironed down to a situation where everyone will be, as far as possible, like everyone else. But of course, that is not the implication of democracy: the implication of democracy is rather that the individual can be as highly developed as lies within the possibilities of his own inheritance, and still can enter into the attitudes of the others whom he affects (Mead, 1934, p. 326).

Mead and Dewey were both professors at the University of Chicago, and it was in Chicago in the 1920's and 1930's that a whole group of ecological studies were spawned, including the forerunner of a series on mental illness in the community, Faris and Dunham's *Mental Disorders in Urban Areas* (1939).

ADVANCES IN MENTAL-HEALTH TREATMENT, LEGISLATION, AND THEORY

So much for the deeper philosophical and historical roots which underlie the current revolution in mental health. In the more immediate past, the past twenty years, we can identify major advances in treatment, legislation, and theory which have given these roots sustenance and produced new mental-health forms and functions. In 1952, Delay and Denker used ataraxic drugs in Paris, initiating a biochemical-treatment method which has reduced the number of patients in our hospitals and has made community treatment increasingly possible (Cole et al., 1966; Joint Commission on Mental Illness and Health, 1961; Adelson & Epstein, 1962). A year later, in 1953, the publication of Maxwell Jones's *Therapeutic Community* brought a new social-treatment advance, the implementation of which had been made possible by the new drugs. And in 1954, the United States Supreme Court school-desegregation decision *(Brown* v. *Board of Education),* signaled the beginning of an era of community and personal action and development which appeared to have the most profound implications for mental health and self-development, but which also fell clearly outside the medical or treatment model.

Personality and psychological theory was also changing during this period. In 1947, Fromm's *Man for Himself* appeared, with its contrasts of the "marketing" and "productive" orientations and its insistent criticism that psychiatry had become a tool to manipulate man, to help him adjust to prevailing values, instead of a method to help him grow in relation to more universal values. And in 1950 came Erik Erikson's *Childhood and Society,* which described the phases from basic trust to ultimate integrity in individual development.

These two problems, of values and of identity, lie at the core of the current crisis and revolution in mental health. They touch on relations between professionals and the larger community they serve, between the professionals and the patient or client population, between professional and professional, and between the professional and himself. Together with the advances in treatment mentioned above, these problems are having a profound effect on the medical model. And they are also bringing to the fore a new "growth" or "human-potentials" model which has an image of man as a free and responsible being, active in concert with his fellows in bringing about a saner world.

MAJOR EMPHASES OF COMMUNITY MENTAL HEALTH

What are the implications of these scientific advances and of the democratic philosophy for a concept of comprehensive community mental health? Elsewhere (Adelson, 1964a) I have suggested that community mental health appears to me to have the following emphases:

1. The focus on a preventive approach, with a spectrum of community mental-health services.

2. The focus on processes at levels beyond the individual one-to-one relationship: the group process, community-organization process, administrative process, research process, and mental-health-education process, as well as mental-health-consultation process.

3. The new kinds of treatment facilities—community mental-health centers, day and night centers, halfway houses, threshold clubs, and sheltered workshops—all providing bridges for remaining in, or moving back into, the community.

4. The new treatment methods: the therapeutic community, family therapy, multiple-impact therapy, group therapy with various kinds of groups, brief therapy, and crisis intervention.

5. The highly developed community mental-health services with the "caretakers" or "gatekeepers" (welfare workers, police, teachers) who are already working with the larger populations-at-risk for this reason are now called indirect services.

6. The shifting emphasis to increasingly comprehensive and continuous services going hand in hand with greater individualization of the patient.

7. The growing openness of the hospital to the community, and the idea of "one door" with all services viewed as alternatives in the patient's care.

8. The increasingly interdisciplinary nature of work in the field of mental health at both the research and practice levels.

9. The increasing emphasis on research and epidemiological investigation.

10. The increasing incorporation of concepts from such fields as

social psychology, sociology, and anthropology, and their integration with clinical knowledge and insight, giving us a better understanding of social phenomena.

11. The focus on such social systems as the group, the family, the school, the organization, the hospital, and the industry as basic units in the larger community and thus of interest to community mental health.

12. The increasing acceptance of planned change within the framework of the democratic idea.

While these characterize the general trends in this new movement, the form and focus they are given as they are developed over time will depend on whether they are conceived as falling only within the bounds of a traditional-treatment model or also within a growth-and-development model. The following section outlines some of the differences between these models—a polarization with may smack somewhat of a "good guys" and "bad guys" dichotomy, but which is intended as a differentiating step on the way to the reintegration and reconstruction of theory and practice we are seeking.[3] Furthermore, I suggest that a comprehensive program of community mental health must incorporate both models as twin foci.

Traditional-Treatment Model *or* Growth-and-Development Model

The "traditional treatment" is a medical model; the "growth and development" is a social-psychological, economic-political, biological-treatment model. The physician's focus is the mind-body, and his goal is *mens sana in corpore sano*—"a sound mind in a sound body." There is strength in this position, a strength which has been considerably bolstered by the biochemical breakthroughs in psychiatry during the past fifteen years. And the medical-treatment model may, indeed, largely suffice for problems of secondary and tertiary prevention. The growth model is concerned more broadly with men as citizens, *mens sana in corpore sano in civitate sano* —"a sound mind in a sound body in a sound society"—with men in interrelationship in a variety of community subsystems. Evi-

[3]The contrast between "traditional-treatment model" and "growth-and-development model" is an expanded version of a position statement originally prepared for the Boston Conference on the Education of Psychologists for Community Mental Health, May, 1965.

dence has accumulated that such social, economic, and political factors as conditions of work (French et al., 1962; Kornhauser, 1965), unemployment, social class (Srole et al., 1962), community disintegration (Leighton et al., 1963), and minority membership (Clark & Clark, 1947; Kardiner & Ovesey, 1951) all appear related to serious mental- and even physical-health conditions. This is evidence based, for the most part, on research carried out by social scientists not confined by the medical-treatment model. It suggests that at the primary level of prevention at least, there is a total gestalt of processes and conditions beyond the medical which are of fundamental importance. And it raises the question as to whether the medical-treatment model is appropriate or sufficient for dealing with these conditions, at either the theoretical or the practical level.

Doctor-Patient Relationship at Core *or* the Community, Its Social Systems and Its Individuals, at Core

The treatment model has the doctor-patient relationship implicit at its core. This relationship is one of healer to sick or wounded, or of expert or specialist to passive recipient. The problem is that while such a relationship may be necessary and helpful in many instances (see Bergin, 1966) when applied to the "mentally ill," it may produce and/or maintain the very antithesis of the "independence" or "interdependence" which is a criterion of good mental health. On the other hand, when the individual in his family, work, or neighborhood systems participates with others on an egalitarian basis, in pursuit of common goals, he may indeed be moving toward the self-fulfillment and contribution to the community which are essential to positive mental health. Research and practice with a variety of community subsystems—the family (Clausen, 1966), the school (Glidewell et al., 1966), the hospital (Stanton & Schwartz, 1954), the neighborhood (Thelen, 1954), and others (Duhl, 1963)—are teaching us much about conditions beyond the medical which are conducive to good mental health.

Community Defined as Geographic, Territorial, Political Unit *or* as "System of Systems" and as "Common Destiny"

Where the focus is on the patient seen independently by the doctor, community tends to be defined merely as the locale from which patients are drawn or for which agencies are responsible—

a geographic or political unit. The individual seen in relation to the community defined as a "system of systems," suggests that the individual is in dynamic interrelationship in a system. And the theories and concepts of such sociologists as Tönnies (1957), Durkheim (1951), and Parsons (1951) and of such social psychologists as Mead (1934), Lewin (1948), Lippitt (Lippitt et al., 1958), Sarbin (1954), and French (French et al., 1962), among others, add a new dimension to thinking and move the focal center away from treatment and toward prevention and growth.

In our time we have increased our understanding of the significance of community—of the family, the peer group, the work group, and what Cooley (1962) has called "the primary group" for identity. More and more, man is planning and organizing specialized "small communities" as both instruments and ways of life in relation to varied needs. Thus, in the psychiatric world, we have seen the creation of special therapy groups and of therapeutic communities, of such transitional communities as day and night hospitals, halfway houses, threshold clubs, Recovery, Inc.—special communities providing rules, regulations, standards, values, and opportunities for problem solving and for shaping one's self-identity.

The past several decades have also seen the rise of a variety of groups or communities such as Alcoholics Anonymous, Synanon, Tops, Colostomy Clubs, Laryngectomy Clubs, and a variety of other groups which individuals have organized themselves to meet their own needs, so that they have come to be known as self-help groups. Some of us have been impressed by what often appears to be the greater effectiveness of such groups when contrasted with traditional approaches.

And, finally, we have seen the continued proliferation of the voluntary associations which De Tocqueville considered the heart of democracy—associations organized along ethnic, religious, nationality, professional, recreational, and other lines. If, with the breakup of the traditional small community has come the anxiety, which is a concomitant of "freedom from," this has opened the possibility of "freedom to," in Erich Fromm's phrase. If the city has left us alienated, it has also, in the great variety of communities and groups which have developed within its boundaries, provided much greater opportunity for choice of identity. As Portnoy has pointed out in his discussion of anxiety states:

This is a period characterized further by the undermining of many of the basic values, definitions, standards, beliefs, and illusions which previously provided the foundation for man's orientation to himself, to others, and to life. The passing of the age of the powerful "fathers" has left the "sons" (and may we add, "daughters") free to make their own way (Portnoy, 1959, p. 307).

Atomistic Consideration of Individuals, with Focus on Intrapsychic Factors *or* Emphasis on Interrelations between Individuals and Subsystems of Which They Form a Part

The concepts when individuals alone are considered tend to be focused on intrapsychic factors, such as id, ego, and superego. Concepts when systems are considered (von Bertalanffy, 1966) move us to a consideration of such aspects as system boundaries, open and closed systems, roles, statuses, barriers to communication, structure, leadership, atmosphere, cohesiveness, intra- and intersystem relationships (Cartwright & Zander, 1960), and a variety of other variables which social and behavioral scientists have developed to further our understanding of the relations of individuals to society. A number of new practices and approaches have been developed over the past decade which reflect these concerns with a total system: therapeutic community (M. Jones, 1953; Rapoport, 1960; Wilmer, 1958), family therapy (Satir, 1964), multiple-impact therapy (MacGregor et al., 1966), sensitivity training (Bradford et al., 1964), among others.

Psychiatrist and Parapsychiatric Professions with Emphasis on Practice *or* Various Kinds of Scientists and Practitioners Contributing to Community Research and Practice on an Equal Base

In the treatment model, the contribution of the nonmedical professionals on the team is relatively peripheral; they are ancillary to the prime mover—the physician. The social-behavioral sciences are utilized for a broader understanding of factors influencing the core medical model. In the growth model, all professionals meet on an equal base: social scientists, physical scientists and practitioners, nurses, social psychologists, social workers, community organizers, clinical psychologists. It may even be suggested that in this model, the larger population being served is recog-

nized as the ultimate source of authority for the particular compe-
tencies offered by each of the "professional" disciplines in the
process of solving the "community-individual" problems. Ultimately, this kind of shared responsibility may be a *sine qua non*
of mental health. As I have pointed out elsewhere:

In a recent series of visits to a variety of mental health programs in the
country, I was struck by the fact that where traditional one-to-one psychotherapy and psychoanalysis were still emphasized, the nurse continued to
play an extremely traditional role as handmaiden to the psychiatrist.
Where the new treatment methods and new indirect services were used
increasingly, the nurse performed these functions on an equal base with
the other professionals on the team. In the new Chicago zonal centers,
each entering patient may be provided with crisis intervention, individual psychotherapy, group psychotherapy, or family therapy by any of the
professionals, including the nurse. The same is true for the psychiatric
service at Maimonides Hospital in Brooklyn where the nurse participates
in all aspects of patient care and treatment, from intake, diagnostic work-
up, to community organization work and multiple impact therapy when
this is indicated. In the San Mateo, California, Mental Health Program, the
nurse serves as a mental health consultant along with other professionals,
and in the Berkeley Mental Health Program, she is responsible for planning the coordination of aftercare services for individuals discharged
from the hospital, for carrying out pilot surveys of areas in the community
from which patients come, as a guide to planning of services, and for
arranging home visits and family therapy (Adelson, 1969, p. 290).

Goal to Keep Psychiatric Disorders at a Minimum
or Goal to Foster "Growth"

The medical man is usually called upon for the treatment of
specific psychiatric disorders. There is, at the primary level of
prevention, a larger goal, which is to create the conditions and
processes which will foster the growth of all. The growth-and-
development model has the concomitant goal to explore the conditions which impede or stimulate such growth. To this end, the
base in research is on "normal" growth processes and the social
systems which influence these. Is there any alternative to prevention apart from growth—physical, cognitive, emotional, and social? Here I tend to agree with MacKinnon and Maslow:

Most important for motivation and value-theory is the introduction of a
positive force to supplement the Freudian pessimism and the neo-behavioristic relativism. . . . What such a positive concept can do for psychology
is seen in the numerous writings of [Carl] Rogers . . . and his students, in

which the concept of "growth" (indistinguishable from self-actualization) assumes more and more a central and essential role. This can be equally so for a psychological theory of democracy, of interpersonal relations, of social improvement, of cross-cultural comparison, and of a scientific system of values (MacKinnon & Maslow, 1951, p. 646).

Emphasis on Program Evaluation and Assessment of Psychiatric Needs and Resources *or* Emphasis on Research on Relationship of Individual to Groups and to Community

In the medical model and models currently based on it, just as the physician provides medicine, so casework or counseling or group work or occupational therapy is provided as a service; and agencies tend to be caught up in attempts to provide enough services to meet the variety of needs presented by their clients. There follows a demand for evaluation of these programs to test whether they are meeting the needs and how effectively they are doing so on the basis of a variety of criteria. In essence, research again turns around the doctor-patient or caseworker-client relationship. In the growth-and-development model, the individual in relation to his social systems is studied for insights and understandings which may lead to social action as well as to individual treatment. For example, the research done by social scientists on the effects of prejudice became part of the evidence which the United States Supreme Court weighed in the school-desegregation decision of 1954.

Processes Seen in Relation to Doctor-Patient Relationship *or* in Relation to Community and Its Subsystems

In the traditional model, "community organization," for example, is more related to the organization of agencies and services in relation to psychiatric disorders and is closer to the organization of professionals. In the growth-and-development model, "community organization" is at the grass-roots level, as in urban redevelopment or community development. As another example, in the traditional model, "mental-health consultation" offered to nonpsychiatric agencies and professionals tends to be concerned with helping individuals to become more objective, understanding, and insightful with respect to their interpersonal or system problems. In the growth-and-development model, "consultation" is more concerned with effecting system changes related to individual growth.

The power in the traditional medical model remains in the hands of the physician or professional workers. Community organization is from above, often with specific projects in mind (for example, new facilities for mentally retarded children). In the growth model, the development of everyone in the community is of concern, and the conditiòns under which such development can best be fostered are explored. Here we deal with the question of "power over people" via social status, economic, political, or other means—power responded to out of fear as contrasted with the power of shared responsibility and shared decision making and with the significance of these kinds of processes for individual growth and self-esteem (as in the Haryou or Mobilization for Youth projects).

Emphasis on Freudian, Psychoanalytic, and Neo-Freudian Intrapsychic Factors *or* Emphasis on Social and Community Psychological Factors

Theory will not be so different, but the emphasis will move from an orientation on intrapsychic factors to an orientation on social and community psychological factors, as exemplified in the work of Dewey, Mead, Durkheim, Fromm, Lewin, Lippitt, Rogers, and others. The shift in emphasis may be symbolized by a movement away from "lying on the couch" passivity toward a demand for civil-rights and civil-liberties participation and activity. At the base is the democratic process and the notion that, ultimately, the power lies in the people. There is a growing body of behavioral-science research demonstrating the significance for good mental health of democratic leadership and of participation in the democratic process.

It is not insignificant that a major milestone in the experimental literature of group dynamics is also a milestone in the extension of our understanding of the positive effects of democracy at the human-relations level. In their classic study, Lewin, Lippitt, and White (1939) demonstrated the superiority of democratic leadership over authoritarian or laissez-faire leadership. Under democracy there were stronger work motivation and greater originality; under autocracy there were more submissive behavior, less varied conversation, more destruction of property, more demands for attention, more hostility, and more scapegoat behavior. Under laissez-faire there were less and poorer work, more complaints, and more play-minded conversation. As White and Lippitt have pointed out more recently (1960), democracy is almost universally defined as having four characteristics: majority rule, freedom, responsibility, and the safeguarding of individual rights. Moreover, it is freedom with order—neither freedom without order (which may lead to anarchy) nor order without freedom (which may lead to autocracy). The democratic leader does not play a hands-off role, but is active in stimulating group discussion and group decisions.

That active participation in civic and community affairs is associated with higher self-esteem has been shown by Rosenberg (1965) in his study of the self-image of 5,000 adolescents in New York State. A number of investigators (for example, Freedman, 1966) have suggested that the civil-rights movement has resulted in a shifting of energies from aggressive behavior (which may lead to arrest) to behavior which has positive goals for social change (resulting in fewer arrests for criminal offenses) and which, by inference, suggests the positive effects of participation in the democratic process. That the democratic process and participation also have positive effects in a treatment setting has been shown by Hoover and Shulman (1964) in their evaluation of a Veterans Administration hospital which used a guided-democracy approach.

The democratic idea also has been at the core of thought and practice in the therapeutic community as developed by Maxwell Jones (1953), Wilmer (1958), and Bierer (1964), among others. Of interest is Gary Marx's (personal communication) finding that Negroes who are participants in the struggle for civil rights are also those who are least antiwhite in their attitudes.

Focus on the History of the Individual
or on the History of the Community

While individual histories remain important, men who see themselves as related to and carrying a responsibility for their fellow men gain a sense of identity by being aware of their historical relation to the past, the present, and the future and by their sense of "shared destiny" with the community of which they are members. Identity and community are intimately related to each other, and a knowledge of the history of the community provides a sense of perspective and roots for individuals participating in the community's ongoing life and an anchor in times of crisis, as Bettelheim's (1947) discussion of concentration-camp experiences has pointed up.

Diagnosis, Treatment, and Rehabilitation (Secondary and Tertiary Prevention) *or* Commitment and Identity (Primary Prevention)

It follows from the emphases described above that, in the growth model, prevention is ultimately concerned with providing so strong a sense of inner identity and commitment that life's blows and vagaries fall lightly. How such ego strength is developed should be a primary task of research for the community mental-health investigator. Those who are practicing with the traditional model are also interested in this problem, but to their tents come the wounded from life's battlefields. Since there are many such, the traditionalists must perforce devote most of their time, energy, and thought to "treating" these "mind-body" problems.

"Mind-Body" Problems Defining the Boundaries of Concern, with "Social Engineering" Frowned Upon *or* Planned Social and Individual Change within a Democratic Framework

The question of how to effect both social and individual change and growth as a primary means of preventing mental illness is, of all issues, probably the most important. The criteria suggested as a basis for selecting and judging measures and methods to be used are broadly the criteria which are safeguarded by our Constitution and interpreted in our laws and courts. These are the criteria by which the majority rules, with respect for minority rights, with freedom and responsibility seen as interrelated, with means as important as ends, and with the ultimate value on human dignity and respect. Freedom of speech, freedom of the press, freedom of association, and freedom of religion; the right to vote; the separation of church and state are all values based on this ultimate value of the dignity of man.

While the laws and regulations defining the democratic process have evolved over many hundreds of years, what should be noted is that in our time we are coming better and better to understand what may be called the nature of the democratic process at the psychological and social-psychological levels.

Bennis and Shepard (1961) have traced the major phases through which a group and the individuals within the group move: from dependence through counterdependence to resolution and acceptance of individual responsibility after the leader has been symbolically rejected, as the authority and power-relations problem is resolved; and from enchantment through disenchantment to consensual validation, as the interpersonal and acceptance-by-peers problem is resolved. These phases, observed for the sensitivity group, have been found to have relevance in the supervision of social workers (Edelson, 1964), in mental-health consultation (Adelson & Jacobs, 1964), and in the development of a ward group (Kazzaz, 1964).

This is a theory which helps us understand better that group and community development—whether of mentally ill patients as in Sivadon's (1959) work in Paris or in slum areas as in Lurie's (1963) work in East Harlem—may have to go through a stage of rejection of established leadership under one form and its reacceptance under another. Failure to understand this as a necessary phase may cause professional leaders to react with threat and punitiveness, prolonging the dependence and submissiveness which they are trying to overcome.

Kurt Lewin, the father of group dynamics, has also in a variety of experiments clarified the relation between restraining and driving forces at the psychological level in planned change and the significance of the group as a base for changing attitudes and behavior. Most simply put, it would appear that change which is growth-oriented and group-oriented arouses many fewer resistances than does change which is individually oriented and implicitly critical of current practices, whether in work with highly trained professionals (Adelson, 1964a) or with the unskilled and uneducated (Riessman et al., 1964).

CONCLUSION: TWO DILEMMAS AND A QUESTION

I would like, in conclusion, to touch on two dilemmas that we face as human beings and as professionals. In his classic study of Negro-white relations, Gunnar Myrdal (1944) spoke of "an American dilemma," to indicate the disparity between our ideals and our practices. This, I have come to see as the historical human dilemma, whether we speak of the tension between self-ideal and self in actuality, of the relations between man and man, or of the affairs between nation and nation.

As professionals, we are faced also with a constant acceleration of scientific knowledge juxtaposed with countless problems needing solution. The dilemma is how to keep up with the new knowledge and also prepare to make some further contribution. These are not unrelated dilemmas. Scientific advances make more possible the actualization of the democratic ideal; democratic advances increase the numbers of those who can participate meaningfully in the scientific as well as the democratic enterprise.

Finally, I would like to raise the question which should really have been posed at the beginning in the current identity crisis which those of us in the mental-health field are experiencing: What is mental health? That great contemporary social philosopher-psychiatrist Erich Lindemann has given us a brief, but penetrating definition which, I believe, has relevance for us here: "Mental health appears to demand free commitment to an endeavor in terms of objectives shared within a reference group" (Lindemann, 1963, p. 6).

We have returned to the paradox that freedom is not freedom without bounds. The self-actualizing psyche needs the goals, values, and standards provided by the *self-actualizing community*. Indeed, we need our colleagues to preserve our own individualities. For it is another aspect of this paradox that "only as the individual in society struggles to preserve his individuality in common cause with his fellows can he hope to remain an individual" (Krech et al., 1962, p. 529).

REFERENCES

Adelson, D. The program of the Center for Training in Community Psychiatry and the role of psychologists in its development. Paper presented at symposium of California State Psychological Association, Los Angeles, 1964. (a)

Adelson, D. Research in community psychiatry. In L. Bellak (Ed.), *Handbook of community psychiatry and community mental health.* New York: Grune & Stratton, 1964. (b)

Adelson, D. Community mental health: a new frontier. In M. E. Kalkman (Ed.), *Psychiatric nursing.* (3rd ed.) New York: McGraw-Hill, 1969.

Adelson, D., & Epstein, L. J. A study of phenothiazines with male and female chronically ill schizophrenic patients. *J. nerv. ment. Dis.*, 1962, 134, 543-554.

Adelson, D., & Jacobs, S. Some aspects of mental health consultation with groups. Paper presented at symposium of American Psychological Association, Los Angeles, 1964.

Bellak, L. (Ed.) *Handbook of community psychiatry and community mental health.* New York: Grune & Stratton, 1964.

Bennis, W. G., & Shepard, H. A theory of group development. In W. G. Bennis, K. D. Benne, & R. Chin (Eds.), *The planning of change: readings in the applied behavioral sciences.* New York: Holt, Rinehart & Winston, 1961.

Bergin, A. E. Some implications of psychotherapy research for therapeutic practice. *J. abnorm. Psychol.*, 1966, 71 (4), 235-246.

Bertalanffy, L. von. General system theory and psychiatry. In S. Arieti (Ed.), *American handbook of psychiatry.* Vol. 3. New York: Basic Books, 1966.

Bettelheim, B. Individual and mass behavior in extreme situations. In T. M. Newcomb & R. L. Hartley (Eds.), *Readings in social psychology.* New York: Holt, 1947.

Bierer, J. The Marlborough experiment. In L. Bellak (Ed.), *Handbook of community psychiatry and community mental health.* New York: Grune & Stratton, 1964.

Bradford, L., Gibb, J., & Benne, K. (Eds.) *T-group theory and laboratory method.* New York: Wiley, 1964.

Caplan, G. *Principles of preventive psychiatry.* New York: Basic Books, 1964.

Cartwright, D., & Zander, A. (Eds.) *Group dynamics: research and theory.* Evanston, Ill.: Row, Peterson, 1960.

Clark, K. B., & Clark, M. P. Racial identification and preference in Negro children. In T. M. Newcomb & R. L. Hartley (Eds.), *Readings in social psychology.* New York: Holt, 1947.

Clausen, J. A. Family structure, socialization and personality. In L. W. Hoffman & M. L. Hoffman (Eds.), *Review of child development research.* Vol. 2. New York: Russell Sage Foundation, 1966.

Cole, J. O., Goldberg, S. C., & Davis, J. M. Drugs in the treatment of psychosis: controlled studies. In P. Solomon (Ed.), *Psychiatric drugs.* New York: Grune & Stratton, 1966.

Cooley, C. H. *Social organization.* New York: Schocken Books, 1962.

Dewey, J. *Democracy and education.* New York: Macmillan, 1916.

Dewey, J. Psychology and social practice. Reprinted in J. Ratner (Ed.), *J. Dewey: philosophy, psychology and social practice.* New York: Putnam, 1963.

Duhl, L. J. (Ed.) *The urban condition.* New York: Basic Books, 1963.

Durkheim, E. *Suicide.* Glencoe, Ill.: Free Press, 1951.

Edelson, Marjory. The utilization of group process in social work supervision. Unpublished manuscript, 1964.

Erikson, E. *Childhood and society.* New York: Norton, 1950. (2nd ed., 1963)

Faris, R. E. L., & Dunham, W. H. *Mental disorders in urban areas: an ecological study of schizophrenia and other psychoses.* Chicago: Univer. of Chicago Press, 1939.

Frank, Sister Charles M. *The historical development of nursing.* Philadelphia: Saunders, 1953.

Freedman, L. Z. Psychiatry and the law. In *Progress in neurology and psychiatry.* Vol. 21. New York: Grune & Stratton, 1966.

French, J. P. R., Kahn, R. L., & Mann, F. C. Work, health and satisfaction. *J. soc. Issues,* 1962, **18** (3).

Fromm, E. *Man for himself.* New York: Rinehart, 1947.

Gardner, J. W. *Excellence.* New York: Harper & Row, 1962.

Glidewell, J. C., Kantor, M. B., Smith, L. M., & Stringer, L. A. Socialization and social structure. In L. W. Hoffman & M. L. Hoffman (Eds.), *Review of child development research.* Vol. 2. New York: Russell Sage Foundation, 1966.

Goodman, P., & Goodman, P. *Communitas.* (2nd ed.) New York: Vintage Books, 1960.

Hoover, K. K., & Shulman, B. H. Therapeutic democracy: some changes in staff-patient relationships. Paper presented at the First International Congress of Socail Psychology, London, 1964. Published in *J.soc. Psychiat.* (Special Edition No. 3), August 1964, pp. 16–23.

Howe, Louisa P. The concept of the community. In L. Bellak (Ed.), *Handbook of community psychiatry and community mental health.* New York: Grune & Stratton, 1964.

Joint Commission on Mental Illness and Health. *Action for mental health.* New York: Basic Books, 1961.

Jones, E. *The life and work of Sigmund Freud.* Vol. 2. New York: Basic Books, 1955.

Jones, M. *Therapeutic community.* New York: Basic Books, 1953.

Kardiner, A., & Ovesey, L. *The mark of oppression: explorations in the personality of the American Negro.* New York: Norton, 1951.

Kazzaz, D. The development of a psychiatry team in the light of a group development theory. *J. of Fort Logan ment. Hlth Center,* 1964, 2, 101-115.

Kornhauser, A. *Mental health and the industrial worker.* New York: Wiley, 1965.

Krech, D., Crutchfield, R., & Ballachey, E. *Individual in society: a textbook of social psychology.* New York: McGraw-Hill, 1962.

Leighton, Dorothea C., Harding, J. S., Macklin, D. B., Macmillan, A. M., & Leighton, A. H. *The character of danger: psychiatric symptoms in selected communities.* New York: Basic Books, 1963.

Lewin, K., Lippitt, R., & White, R. K. Patterns of aggressive behavior in experimentally created "social climates." *J. soc. Psychol.,* 1939, 10, 291–279.

Lindemann, E. Mental health and the environment. In L. J. Duhl (Ed.), *The urban condition.* New York: Basic Books, 1963.

Lippitt, R., Watson, J., & Westley, B. *The dynamics of planned change.* New York: Harcourt, Brace, 1958.

Lippitt, R. O., & White, R. K. An experimental study of leadership and group life. In T. M. Newcomb & R. L. Hartley (Eds.), *Readings in social psychology.* New York: Holt, 1947.

Lurie, Ellen. Community action in East Harlem. In L. J. Duhl (Ed.), *The urban condition.* New York: Basic Books, 1963.

MacGregor, R., Ritchie, A. M., Serrano, A. C., Schuster, F. P., Jr., McDanald, E. C., & Goolishian, H. A. *Multiple impact therapy with families.* New York: McGraw-Hill, 1966.

MacKinnon, D. W., & Maslow, A. H. Personality. In H. Helson (Ed.), *Theoretical foundations of psychology.* New York: Van Nostrand, 1951.

Mead, G. H. *Mind, self, and society: from the standpoint of a social behaviorist.* Chicago: Univer. of Chicago Press, 1934.

Myrdal, G. *An American dilemma: the Negro problem and modern democracy.* New York: Harper, 1944.

Parsons, T. *The social system.* Glencoe, Ill.: Free Press, 1951.

Portnoy, I. The anxiety states. In S. Arieti (Ed.), *American handbook of psychiatry.* Vol. 1. New York: Basic Books, 1959.

Rapoport, R. N. *Community as doctor.* London: Tavistock, Thomas, 1960.

Riessman, F., Cohen, J., & Pearl, A. *Mental health of the poor.* New York: Free Press of Glencoe, 1964.

Rosenberg, M. *Society and the adolescent self-image.* Princeton, N.J.: Princeton Univer. Press, 1965.

Sarbin, T. Role theory. In G. Lindzey (Ed.), *Handbook of social psychology.* Vol. 1. *Theory and method.* Cambridge, Mass.: Addison-Wesley, 1954.

Satir, Virginia. *Conjoint family therapy.* Palo Alto, Calif.: Science and Behavior Books, 1964.

Sivadon, P. D. Techniques of sociotherapy. In Mabel Cohen (Ed.), *Advances in psychiatry.* New York: Norton, 1959.

Smith, M. B., & Hobbs, N. *The community and the community mental health center.* Washington, D.C.: Amer. Psychological Association, 1966.

Srole, L., Langner, T. S., Michael, S. T., Opler, M. K., & Rennie, T. A. C. *Mental health in the metropolis: the midtown Manhattan study.* New York: McGraw-Hill, 1962.

Stanton, A. H., & Schwartz, M. S. *The mental hospital: a study of institutional participation in psychiatric illness and treatment.* New York: Basic Books, 1954.

Thelen, H. *The dynamics of groups at work.* Chicago: Univer. of Chicago Press, 1954.

Thompson, M. M. *The history of education.* New York: Barnes & Noble, 1953.

Tönnies, F. *Community and society.* New York: Harper & Row, 1957.

White, R. K., & Lippitt, R. O. *Autocracy and democracy.* New York: Harper, 1960.

White, R. W. *The abnormal personality.* New York: Ronald Press, 1948.

Wilmer, H. A. *Social psychiatry in action.* Springfield, Ill.: Thomas, 1958.

CHAPTER 2

The Commitment of Community Psychology

William C. Rhodes

The recent positions taken by the American Psychological Association with respect to the community mental-health centers and private health insurance are probably the first major public utterances and social stances released to the mass audience by our guild. This is one form of commitment; it is a guild commitment to a common guild stance.

As a psychologist who has suffered many limitations and frustrations at the hands of medicine and psychiatry, I applaud this type of commitment. But I know that my applause is based upon the desire to have the same type of clout behind *me* and *my* actions as the psychiatrist has had behind his. It is based upon the release of long-pentup anger and resentment at having to work in medically dominated structures because they were the only channels into the psychological problems of the human community.

Nevertheless, despite the significance of these position statements, and despite my support for them, I wonder if this is what is meant by *commitment.* For one thing, it is probable that the encapsulated professional guild system has reached its peak and either is on the decline or will be supplanted by a consortium form of professionalism. The days in which the operating agencies both supported the strength of the guilds and were more or less captives of single guilds may be on the way out. The old-line single-guild agencies and operational patterns are being supplemented rapidly with operational patterns which cut across guild lines, such as some of the poverty programs, housing and urban-affairs programs, and the like.

We will probably soon see many other types of amalgamated operational patterns, in which a number of professions or a number of agencies come together under a common umbrella to tackle the multiple nature of human ecological problems. These kinds of organizations and programs will not support the type of guild control we have known up to now.

Even more important, the tenor of the times cannot tolerate the partitioning off of human problems into guild jurisdictions and guild territories. It cannot support the ownership of a body of knowledge, a program of training and indoctrination, and a set of technologies by a single guild. Psychology cannot continue to own the body of knowledge of the science of psychology, nor can education continue to own the methods of teaching, nor psychiatry the methods of psychotherapy. Nor can any of these professional systems stake out their claim to special functional qualities of the human organism, as medicine has done in the case of the biological-physical functioning of people whom they claimed as "patients," or as education has done in the case of the vast area of learning by monopolizing "pupils."

There is a dukedom or fiefdom quality about such hard-structured power-political arrangements for regulating the interchange between individuals and their various community environments. The established agencies have built strong political power bases in the community by tying themselves to their own militant guild forces on one side and to political patronage and political protectorates on the other.

THE NEED FOR NEW SOCIAL SOLUTIONS

There are two major reasons why we will have to find quite different social-systems solutions to the problems of human ecology. The first reason is that our human ecological sciences are beginning to collect an impressive array of evidence about the interrelated or gestalt nature of human-community dysfunctioning. Witness human dysfunctioning in its natural ecological setting: problems do not neatly partition themselves off in counterpoint to the partitioned jurisdictions of the political-guild/agency interlocks which have been created for their regulation. The intermingling with the human skin and within the living human groups of such problems as the economic, medical-physical, psychological, and educational defies our ability to differentiate them in the same neat packages as those at the agencies.

The second reason why we will have to find quite different kinds of social-systems solutions to the problems of human ecology lies in the sweeping psychosocial upheavals which are taking place across the country. We are in a fluid historical period in which there is profound repositioning of human claims and rights vis-à-vis social claims and rights. This situation is creating pressure for change in the established ecology-regulator agencies such as education, social welfare, legal correction, mental health, and so forth.

A NEW PSYCHOLOGICAL ERA

The civilizing process conducted through this established ecology-regulation apparatus is not effectively modulating the incompatabilities between man and man and between individual claims and social claims.

A symptom of intensifying incompatability is the increasing psychosocial tension arising from the failure of our society to accommodate subcultural groups such as the Negroes, the Puerto Ricans, the Indians, the Appalachians, the Mexican-Americans, the Cajuns. Another symptom is the repeated threat-recoil process arising out of the individual behaviors of the suicidal, the homicidal, the alcoholic, the psychotic, the neurotic, the cultural deviate, the emotionally disturbed, and the retarded.

The dawning realization of both the importance and the inadequacy of our ecology-regulator systems can be seen in the attacks of slum dwellers upon entrenched and institutionalized systems such as schools, welfare departments, and the legal-correctional paraphernalia. There are even internal revolts of personnel within the systems against regulatory rigidities such as those being conducted by nuns and priests against dogmas of the church.

We are witnessing the awakening of man to a new psycho-ecological reality. Man now stands in a new relationship to his world. It is no longer the mere relationship of a physical being to a physical world. Man's psychological dimensions have gained access to community structures, and our ecological situation is moving very fast toward accommodation to his psychological depths and claims. Old patterns of ecology regulation are limited and increasingly ineffective in helping man toward this new relationship to his world.

Man's psychological nature, in its greater depths, has emerged as an insistent part of the whole which refuses any longer to be denied—and which cannot be denied if man is to survive. Prior to this era, the psychological depths could be ignored or transformed or displaced. The multiple facets of our psychological selves which were at variance with the society could be concealed from ourselves and from relevant others. They could be projected into external ecological problems and physical dimensions and struggled with on that plane. Or, as an alternative, we could project our socially troubling urges onto undesirable populations in our midst. Now this is no longer possible. We have begun to recognize ourselves in the rejected others. We have caught glimpses of our own internal quarrels with society in their social defiance or social incompetency.

We have begun to move even beyond the relatively enlightened concepts which held that the man who could not bring the forces of his inner self into balance with the existing social world was either incompetent or sick. We have begun to move beyond insistence upon repression, suppression, and subjugation of vast inner-life areas as a necessary condition for survival in the social world. We now ask that social reality be modified to accommodate greater ranges of our inner being instead of our former disproportionate insistence upon accommodation to social reality.

We are becoming aware that the bomb and the extermination camps were not chance mutants, but that they issued directly from hostilities in our own nature. We are awakening to the fact that the antidote must come from wellsprings of constructive and effectual urges within us.

Part of our inner being, long submerged, is surfacing and pouring out into the environmental content. This new state of existence makes long-controlled, private, personal worlds a part of public life. In this new state, there is an accompanying feeling of anomie and an accompanying mobilization of psychological and community defenses against the emergence.

NEW ATTEMPTS TO MANAGE STRAIN AND STRESS

In this climate of human resurgence and social fluidity, the old approaches to the relief of strains and stresses in the exchange between individuals and their environs appear to be giving way to flexible responses to human problem conditions. The stream of today's psychosocial events refuses to be molded to the older calcified systems of the agency-guild/political interlock which were employed to solve yesterday's problems. Instead, fluid, spontaneous, and ever changing organizations are arising alongside the entrenched agencies and molding themselves to the stream of psychosocial events which are occurring out there in the human community.

Rather than total reliance upon hard-structured solutions, the current trend is toward flexible interaction with the dynamic flux of the human community by organizational groups which have the free-flowing form of the amoeba. Today, organizations focused upon human problems are spawned, grow, and become established elements in the social scene very rapidly. They are loosely arranged and can shift their tactical delivery and target of entry into the human community as rapidly as the changing social scene.

Instead of exclusive reliance upon organizational referents, we professionals are beginning to reverse our field and find our referent point in the changing human condition as it occurs in the living environment. This means that instead of building programs and concepts on the basis of agency needs, we are trying to pattern them after human realities.

Instead of investing all our energies in monolithic agencies like welfare and education, we are diversifying our resources and consigning some of them to multiple chains of minor and major social experiments such as the various poverty programs, the Peace Corps, and special demonstration projects.

Instead of further hardening our professional methods, we are encouraging spontaneous interjections into the problem stream of human events. Social workers, for instance, are no longer relying exclusively upon casework and financial aid, but are improvising organizational methods, demonstrations, and protests. As another example, some of my analytically oriented psychiatric friends are beginning to hail operant procedures and behavioral therapy as examples of their wide range of approaches.

Instead of our former insistence upon ideological purity, we now countenance wide divergences from professional dogma. I took part recently in an international meeting populated primarily by psychiatrists. In my discussion group, a day-long confrontation took place between two subgroups. One firmly defended the medical model, and the other insisted that it must go. I couldn't have been more astounded if I had found myself in a theological group debating whether or not God was dead.

Instead of our former preoccupation with role specification and insistence upon legal definitions of our role, we are allowing role diversification and role experimentation. We see community psychiatrists as educators of the power structure, as influencers of the agency programs, as advocates of the poor, as consultants to the legal-correctional system.

We see, then, reflections in the professional scene—developments and dynamics which mirror the events taking place in the outer psychosocial scene. We are in a period of movement and flux —a period of discovery and recovery in the processes of ecological management, which resonate with the current psychosocial revolution of the human condition.

Therefore, when we now talk about commitment, we are probably talking about the extent to which we are willing and able to capture in our own substantive field the reality of the human situation in which we are immersed. The term "community psychology" is probably only a symbolic umbrella for the beginning reorientation of much of our philosophy, our body of knowledge, our technology, our corps of specialists, and our training programs to the reality of this seething human condition. In addition, as Newbrough suggests in his insightful paper (Chapter 3), it may also become the title of a particular group of specialists within psychology.

THE UNIQUE ADVANTAGES OF THE UNIVERSITY

Be that as it may, I think there is something very prophetic in the fact that many papers address themselves to the changing scene from a university base. There is something ponderous and intractable about long-established agencies. Because of their exposed position, they are much more vulnerable to public, political, and guild pressures for instant solution; and because of the same exposure and pressure, they are much more cautious about experimentation and risk. Their major orientation too often is to organizational maintenance rather than to substantive bodies of knowledge. Their efforts revolve in large measure around expanding their organization and establishing new organizational beachheads. A substantive problem which galvanizes the community into action too often presents a favorable opportunity for organizational expansion. Their probable solution to any new problem or new form of an old problem seems to be to establish another edition of their organizational prototype in the vicinity of the problem.

Universities are in a much better position to experiment with new forms of ecology regulation and new operational patterns tailored to problem conditions. University faculties have the advantage of a solid base in expanding and flexible substantive knowledge. They can create loops between expanding knowledge and social experimentation. Furthermore, they would not have as much vested interest in maintaining any organizational form of social invention which they produce.

It would seem, therefore, that if universities are willing to step into the mainstream of community affairs and place their scholarship, exploration, and research in the living substance of human interactions in the societal body, they would have unique advantages over community agencies in coming to grips with the tenor of the times.

CHAPTER 3

Community Psychology:
A New Specialty in Psychology?

J. R. Newbrough*

The term "community psychology" has begun to find frequent use in psychology. It seems to have originated at Peabody College about 1958 (Newbrough et al., in press) and achieved national prominence at the Boston Conference on the Education of Psychologists for Community Mental Health (Bennett et al., 1966). A Division of Community Psychology was formed within the American Psychological Association in 1966, and a meeting was held at the University of Texas in early 1967 to discuss training programs in community psychology (APA, 1967). It is the purpose of this paper to consider the characteristics of this newly named area to see whether it represents a significant new segmentation in psychology, and, if so, what might be the course of events to be observed.

THE EMERGENCE OF COMMUNITY PSYCHOLOGY

Community psychology seems to be a product of the development of clinical and counseling psychology after World War II and the more recent social legislation which includes mental health, mental retardation, health, poverty, education, and welfare. It has attracted psychologists who have been working with individuals and groups in the community in attempting to solve personal and social problems, to plan for new services, and to evaluate many of

*The author extends his appreciation to D. N. Lloyd, Ann C. Maney, H. J. Ehrlich, H. C. Haywood, F. C. Noble, and G. L. Lawrence for their helpful comments. The paper was originally prepared when the author was on the staff of the Mental Health Study Center, National Institute of Mental Health, Adelphi, Maryland.

the new programs. While they apparently are largely psychologists with clinical training (now dissatisfied with office practice), there was a wide range of training represented in the new APA division (APA, 1966). Interest in the community as the arena of application was stated very strongly (Bennett et al., 1966). The Boston conference also indicated a considerable desire to instigate and carry out change. This would suggest that most individuals in the area are those with interests in applied science.

COMMUNITY PSYCHOLOGY AS
APPLIED PSYCHOLOGY

In order to gain some perspective on this area of community psychology, the development of applied psychology in general will be considered briefly. The history of applied psychology began about the same time as psychology itself, in the late nineteenth century (Fryer & Henry, 1950; Paterson, 1940; Murphy, 1949). This was at a time when the ideas of human and social improvement of the Age of Enlightenment were being incorporated into society (Rosen, 1959). In addition, the philosophy of pragmatism was developing and asserting the relational and utilitarian nature of knowledge. As a reflection of the times, it was only natural that as psychology developed, its ideas, knowledge, and skills would be applied to practical problems. These problems have included studies of learning, clinical diagnosis and remedial treatment of learning problems, identification of the mentally retarded, screening of military recruits, study of individual differences, participation in child guidance, work on problems of industrial organization and production, personnel selection, crime and correction (Fryer & Henry, 1950; Poffenberger, 1942). The list of problems is long; the list of eminent psychologists working on them is equally long (Paterson, 1940).

One way to test whether community psychology ought to be considered an area of applied psychology is to compare the definitions of the two. Poffenberger offered the following statement to describe applied psychology:

The problem of applied psychology is so to adjust differentially endowed individuals by training them, by selection of their environment, and by the control of this environment that they may attain the maximum of social productivity and the maximum of personal satisfaction (Poffenberger, 1942, p. 13).

Compare the preceding with the following statement from the proceedings of the Boston conference:

Community Psychology ... is devoted to the study of general psychological processes that link social systems with individual behavior in complex interactions. ... such linkages were seen as providing the basis for action programs directed toward improving individual, group and social system functioning (Bennett et al., 1966, p. 7).

In both cases, the application of knowledge for the improvement of the present and the future is the goal. Community psychology, however, seems to have moved away from a strictly individual orientation to one of individuals in relationship to social systems. This divergence shows the introduction of sociological concepts (for example, social system) as a basis for explaining behavior.

"Community" in the term "community psychology" may represent something of a misnomer. It seems to have a vague meaning, indicating the place where psychology is to be applied to the problems of people who are to be found there. It does not seem to include the meaning in sociology of a psychological identity based on the sharing of something in common, for example, living area, professional interest, avocation, and the like. Nor is there much attention to the companion concept, alienation, to refer to the estrangement of people from their community, the loss of social control within the community, and their engagement in deviant behavior. There would seem to be a parallel here with the reductionistic approach of physiological psychologists, who see the explanation for behavior in electrical and chemical terms. For the community psychologist, sociological concepts (for example, social organization, social system, power, sanction) provide the explanation and the meaning for behavior. It is these concepts which provide the basis for conceptualizing approaches to the action programs mentioned above. Since they are the language of explanation (for example, "the apathy of these citizens is due to their alienation and lack of social power"), it does not seem to be necessary to go into the elaboration of their meanings as developed by sociological writers. Thus, it would seem that community psychology may refer to the application of sociological concepts by psychologists in their dealing with individual behavior in the community.

COMMUNITY PSYCHOLOGY AS A NEW SPECIALTY IN PSYCHOLOGY

Community psychology is an area of work for psychologists concerned with the application of scientific knowledge to the solution of immediate social problems, such as poverty and education. It is of interest to consider whether the area, as a next step, will develop as a new specialty in psychology and to speculate about the course of its professional development. In order to examine the development, the following discussion will draw on a frame of reference from the sociological study of professions.

Bucher and Strauss (1960-1961) have developed a process model for the analysis of the development of professions. The model goes beyond the view that a profession is relatively homogeneous, unified, and stable to a conception of a profession as a loose amalgamation "of segments pursuing different objectives in different manners and more or less delicately held together under a common name at a particular period in history." Many psychologists would find it easy to apply this statement to psychology.

Using this model, we will consider community psychology as a developing segment of psychology, with discussion under the following topics:

1. Nature of the mission.
2. Type of work performed.
3. Methods and techniques employed.
4. Clients served.
5. Colleagueship.
6. Interests and associations.
7. Relations with the public.[1]

Nature of the Mission

A segment of a profession typically defines a purpose or mission which is unique to it and which is publicly proclaimed as such. The mission often arises out of a struggle for recognition and status within the profession and with the aim of excluding others from the segment. The Boston conference identified the mission of community psychology as broader than community mental health and concerned with programs of social action for the purpose of

---

[1]In the use of the process model for analysis, the general descriptive statements were taken from the Bucher and Strauss (1960-1961) discussion.

effecting social change to improve the life situation of many citizens.

Type of Work Performed

A number of different tasks are performed in the name of the profession. These are accompanied by a variety of ideas about what constitutes the *most important* work. This statement is particularly descriptive of psychology. Within community psychology, the specific work includes diagnosis and treatment of individuals, consultation with community leaders and agency personnel about a variety of problems, development of specific programs (for example, preschool emotional screening of children, mental-health education of parents), research and evaluation of the programs, and training of nonprofessionals. The Boston conference suggested that the areas of consultation and collaboration constitute the major service areas, with the primary work role as that of a "participant–conceptualizer generalist" (Bennett et al., 1966).[2] The conference did not seem to deal clearly with the latent conflict in whether the primary work is service or research. This has been a point of contention since 1917, when the American Association of Applied Psychology split off from the American Psychological Association because the latter was too academic; the conflict reappeared with the formation of the Psychonomic Society in 1959 because the APA was too applied. While the Psychonomic Society was criticizing the APA for its service orientation, the practicing clinical psychologists were attacking the APA for being too academic. This fight generated force and emotion, particularly at the 1964 annual convention of the APA in Los Angeles, and nearly resulted in the formation of other splinter groups (Newbrough, 1964). Community psychology has not been directly part of the service-versus-research struggle, but it may well become an arena for this conflict. The report of the Boston conference emphasized participation in action, but was entirely unclear about the relative importance of action alone as contrasted with participation for the purpose of study. The University of Texas conference in 1967, however, clearly emphasized the prime importance of research. It was a meeting of academics, so perhaps the research emphasis was entirely predictable.

[2]The title was derived from the discussion by Bennett et al. (1966), and did not, as such, appear therein.

Methods and Techniques Employed

The sharpest divisions among members within a profession are thought to be around their choice of methods and techniques. These choices often reflect differences in opinion about the reality with which the profession is concerned. The techniques of individual assessment and psychotherapy have been identified by many as the methods *not* to employ.[3] Not only are such methods believed to be inefficient, but they tend to limit the definition of the problem to an individual. It has become fashionable to extend the limits of the problem to groups of people, to institutions, even to society (Knobel, 1966; Newbrough, 1966a). The purpose of work for the community psychologist has changed from the solution of individual problems to the more general concern with the adjustment of all individuals within a community (Bennett et al., 1966). Research has taken on a more social and environmental flavor (Barker, 1962; Newbrough, 1966a, 1966b). The conceptual framework has become that of systems within systems, all interrelated (Miller, 1965). The "model" for practice proposed at the Boston conference was termed the "educational-learning approach" in contrast with the "disease-treatment approach" to distinguish it from the medical orientation of clinical psychology.

Clients Served

Members of segments of professions become involved in sets of relationships with clients which are distinctive to them. New types of persons may become part of their "work drama." Clinical psychologists deal typically with individuals who have personal problems; in community psychology, citizens of various types and social classes, political leaders, and businessmen have become clients for help with problems common to a number of people, perhaps including themselves. Going beyond this description, some have suggested that the community, or one of its subgroups, is the client (Jacques, 1961; Pages, 1961). Conceiving their work as being within the system of the community, psychologists have begun to regard themselves as secondarily related to individual citizens with problems and primarily related to the "natural agents" within a locality (Kelly, 1964).

---

[3]There is considerable difference of opinion on this point, with some workers believing that case-centered work within a system can provide the basis for indirectly effecting systemic change.

Colleagueship

The sharing of a sense of *esprit* and of kindredness is character-istic of colleagueship and can be a very sensitive indicator of segmentation. The *Proceedings* of the Boston conference contain a sense of excitement and exhilaration among the conferees about direct participation in and influence on the function of the com-munity. There was a shared feeling that social participation and social action are important to community psychologists. The early mailings and the production of an informal newsletter prior to the establishment of the formal division within the APA showed a strong sense of colleagueship and common interest. Perhaps part of the kindredness was a shared sense of leaving the "Model T" techniques of clinical psychology for a new area. The holding of symbols in common is also important in the development of a sense of colleagueship; the choice of the unique term "community psy-chology" may represent the beginning of the symbolization proc-ess.

Interests and Associations

Professionals are described as sharing interests in purpose and goals. Within a profession, however, such interests often diverge and may even be in direct conflict. The areas of conflict seem to be in (1) gaining a proper foothold in institutions, (2) recruitment, and (3) relations to the outside. In order to protect interests and to gain a secure base of operations, specific associations are often formed. The formation of a Division of Community Psychology within the American Psychological Association seems to be an outcome of the intraprofessional conflict—a conflict of broader proportions than community psychology. It has been described as the practitioners seeking recognition and a place of influence within the professional association (Newbrough, 1964). The re-cruitment function requires representation in training centers in order that the segment survive. A number of university training programs are now including courses and field experiences in com-munity psychology or community mental health (APA, 1967). This should serve to provide a place for community psychology within the profession. Relations with the outside have been focused around intra- and interprofessional issues. Within psychology there is debate about whether the trainers of skills in academic settings should not also be practitioners, and whether psychologists need to become fully independent professionals in their own right. These two themes involve the issues of competence and status. Outside the profession, community psychology has considerable interest in common with other social-science and mental-health disciplines. Participants at the Boston conference seemed mainly concerned with separation from medicine and psychiatry and with establishment of an identity. They seemed not to have addressed themselves to relations with other professions except to approve of interdisciplinary training and work. The issues of competence and status will not be solved in community psychology until the matters of a body of knowledge and a separate theoretical orientation have been settled, and until a clearer identity is established.

Relations with the Public

The aspects of a profession for the protection and education of the public (such as a formal association, codes of ethics, and certification) often provide an image to the public of seeming unity with definite characteristics. Internally, these have the effect of controlling the behavior of individuals and segments. They can define what is approved training, what can be certified as advanced professional skills (for example, with diplomas from the American Board of Examiners in Professional Psychology), and what are ethical practices. There has been serious question whether the controlling and constraining forces within the profession will allow for the broader acceptance of applied practitioners into psychology and for the development of new applied specialties. Both the Boston conference in 1965 and the Chicago conference in 1965 (Hoch et al., 1966) supported experimentation in training. Government funding and professional approving agencies are becoming more liberal about what constitutes psychological practice. Within all this, community psychology finds itself advocating training which is at sufficient variance with standard clinical training that some readjustments within the profession will have to be made. At this stage in its development, community psychology as a formal specialty has concerned itself primarily with relations within the profession and not with the general public.

This view of community psychology within the Bucher-Strauss

model would seem to indicate that segmentation of the profession into an area of community psychology is well begun. With the external societal supports in the form of (1) national legislation, (2) national enabling programs of guidance and support, (3) local programs of services, and (4) favorable responses of those being served, all rapidly expanding, one can reasonably predict that the differentiation process will continue.

THE COURSE OF DEVELOPMENT: COUNSELING PSYCHOLOGY AS AN EXAMPLE

In order to predict the possible developmental themes of community psychology as a new psychological specialty, the experience of counseling psychology will be considered. Taking the first national conference as the formal beginning, counseling psychology as a specialty began with the Northwestern conference in 1952 (APA, 1952).[4] Graduate training in counseling and guidance had been ongoing at the universities for many years; the conference was an attempt to establish minimum standards for doctoral-level training and thereby to upgrade the specialty. The issues of concern to counseling for its first six years were reviewed by Berdie (1959) in his presidential address to the Division of Counseling Psychology in 1958. They were:[5]

1. Who determines the purposes of counseling—client or counselor?

2. Are counseling and psychotherapy the same?

3. Is it possible for the counseling process to be unaffected by the counselor's own values?

4. Should counseling be done only by psychologists?

5. Can the counselor's actions be determined by his own professional code of ethics?

6. To what extent does the effectiveness of counseling depend upon sound psychological and social theory?

7. Must counseling always be on a voluntary basis? Can discipline and counseling mix?

The two major themes which seem to run through these issues

[4]This was the same year that Division 17 of the American Psychological Association dropped the word "guidance" from its name and became the Division of Counseling Psychology.

[5]The issues appeared in the original article as "dogma" assertions; they have been recast into questions for this discussion.

are (1) the nature of counseling and how it differs from other activities, and (2) the nature of values and ethics necessary for proper control of counselor work. A review of the *Journal of Counseling Psychology* from 1954 to 1960 indicates a differing development of these two themes. Beginning in 1954 and continuing until 1960, four or five articles per issue were devoted to the theory and process of counseling. Ethics of practice appeared in 1955 in two articles and continued to appear occasionally through 1958. In 1959 and 1960 the question of the counselor's values was featured at symposia at the APA annual meeting with several of the papers also appearing in the journal. What seems to have occurred was initial preoccupation and concern with the establishment of the specialty; the concern with controls began more slowly and continually increased.

It would seem reasonable to predict that community psychology will go through a similar process of differentiation into a specialty. Concern with how it differs will be directed to clinical psychology and social psychology and, to a lesser extent, counseling and school psychology. With its emphasis on social action for social change, the matter of values and ethics may emerge much sooner than they did in counseling. While considerable thought has been given to the matter of ethics in planned social change (Bennis, Benne, & Chin, 1961), the specialty will probably have to fight these battles for itself—much as a child must go through a struggle for identity and values, unable to benefit from the solutions of others. In some way, the segmentation process can be described as a natural course of events which must be played out with the establishment of each professional specialty—with basic themes and issues remaining the same.

THE CONTRIBUTION OF COMMUNITY PSYCHOLOGY

Both Poffenberger (1942) and Gouldner (1961) have observed that in applied science one does not merely apply knowledge derived from the laboratory to natural events. Without the elaborate controls on variables possible in the laboratory, natural situations often yield unpredictable results. Applied science provides the opportunity for the advancement of scientific knowledge and theory, particularly about natural events. To illustrate, Gouldner noted that research on disasters revealed three areas of deficit in pure sociological theory: It had little to say about (1) the role of material props, (2) the relationship between social or cultural systems and the "natural" environment, and (3) the effects of sudden, abrupt change.

Community psychology may have a special role in applied social science, as in applied psychology, in the conduct of research to solve human-relations problems and in the formulation of new knowledge about the natural behavior of individuals and groups. This role is to study the interrelationships of individual, social, and environmental variables in the events and processes of community life. The notion of the "community as a laboratory" was advanced by Klein (1960)* as a frame of reference to illustrate the unique opportunities for naturalistic research available in most community-service programs. This idea was new to psychology and was, in many ways, similar to the development of "ecological" inquiries by sociologists at the University of Chicago in the 1930's (Duncan, 1964). The Chicago research was directed toward the identification of areas in the city which had particular behavioral characteristics. Natural areas were described in their spatial and functional interrelationships to each other, and were viewed as settings in which one could observe behavior resulting from social and ecological processes (Warren, 1963).

The research of psychologists, viewing the community from an ecological perspective, can be expected to elaborate the correlations between environmental and subject variables in the description of naturally observed behavior. To illustrate, a higher frequency of cases of mental disorder from particular areas in Chicago was shown by Faris and Dunham (1939). What has not been clarified is whether this is due to the congregation of particular kinds of people in specific areas, the peculiar effects of the area on people, or the way the area is structured so that certain behavior is more visible in settings where it is likely not to be tolerated or accepted. As another example, consider whether a particular slum is really a bad place to live. And from what perspective? The housing may be bad, but the social supports for people may be strong and functional. The supports may be as much a function of the layout of the houses as the characteristics of the people—a function, for example, of a common backyard with the only water

*Subsequent to this writing, Klein developed the concept more fully. See D. C. Klein, *Community dynamics and mental health* (New York: Wiley, 1968).

faucet in it. Moving the same people as a unit to apartments may as effectively destroy the social supports as relocating them in entirely different areas. Research at an individual and small-group level will help to explain the effects of living in particular settings and should help to bring new data to bear on commonly observed facts and accepted knowledge.

A problem imposed by this orientation is that of idiography; that is, the difficulty of generalizing knowledge from one situation to another. The more detailed and more specific the inquiry, the more unique the knowledge. This factor is what seemed to cause the Chicago research to reach a plateau (Warren, 1963). The question arises as to whether community psychology will be more effective than the Chicago sociologists were in dealing with the idiographic problem. The task will require a line of inquiry which attempts to be idiographic at the level of describing and solving particular problems and, at the same time, nomothetic when extracting principles of use to others. This method has been tried by clinical psychologists and has left them frustrated with their results. The problem may, however, reside as much with their particular training. Community psychology has begun to emphasize field experience and training. If it includes field-research methods and techniques, the training may be sufficient to this continuing challenge.

As an applied area, most of the efforts of community psychology can be expected to be directed toward programs of service. This is because planning and evaluation have become such an important part of contemporary social programs. Health services, mental-health centers, and poverty programs contain provisions for program evaluation; it is to this evaluation that psychologists with their research training are usually asked to apply themselves. The question typically regarded as essential is whether the program has any merit. Research is thought to be the way to answer the question. In order to be clear about the role of research I prefer to describe the research as "program research" and to assign the term "program evaluation" to the judgment made by someone about the worth of the program or services. With this as prologue, it might be helpful to take a broader perspective and to consider the entire process surrounding service programs as "program evolution."

Program evolution is defined as the over-all process of program development, program research, program-relevant background or contextual research, and program evaluation. At any given time, a program lacks what it could ideally reach even in a static situation; given the changing times, this means that the ideal will also be constantly changing. Thus, the critical aspect of any program of service is to provide for its progressive evolution to higher levels of quality and efficiency, The process of inquiry through research applied to practical problems could provide an unbalancing force through a managed conflict between service goals and research findings which could serve to produce change in the organization and in the delivery of services.

Community psychology, with its systems and data-based orientation, can perhaps contribute to the development of programs built on either a feedback or conflict principle which will yield a continuous process of adjustment to new circumstances.

COMMUNITY PSYCHOLOGY: FIELD RESEARCH ON APPLIED PROBLEMS

As a new specialty in psychology, community psychology seems well along the way in the first stages of formation. It can be expected to progress through the stages of identity formation, establishment of an image, and acceptance by psychologists and nonpsychologists alike. Thus, community psychology joins the ranks of a number of areas in applied psychology (for example, clinical, counseling, and school psychology) most of which are themselves undergoing considerable change.

Applied psychology arose from a nineteenth-century science which distinguished between basic and applied orientations (Hunt, 1952). The distinction was based on the purpose of the inquiry: whether it was to solve a practical problem or to add to a body of general knowledge. Each was thought to be somewhat exclusive of the other, with basic research being the highest goal of science. Thus, basic research has had the higher status, both in science and in psychology.

This view has been increasingly questioned as scientists have become more functionalistic in their points of view. As noted earlier, Gouldner (1961) argued that applied research has its own specific characteristics and provides unique opportunities for inquiry. It is not merely basic research taken into the field. Thus, it would seem more accurate to make two distinctions, thinking of them as on unrelated dimensions and making a fourfold table.

There is the *basic-applied* distinction based on the orientation toward problems of immediacy and practicality, and a *laboratory-field* distinction based on where the inquiry gathers its data. Community-psychology practice and research most typically would seem to fall into the *applied, field* cell.

With most of the work of community psychology carried out in the field (the community), it is clear that the primary need for training lies in methods of observation and data gathering. It is interesting to note that the commonality of the community-oriented programs in graduate departments of psychology, as described at the Texas conference, was with field experience and field training. Field work is a matter in common with all applied specialties in psychology and suggests the need for special training in this area. Clinical training has made considerable use of field experience since the Boulder conference in 1949 (Raimy, 1950) so clearly emphasized practice. This has served to highlight the disjunction between service and laboratory research. The major fault with clinical training has been the lack of any training in *field-research methods*. This has been the fault in all areas of applied psychology and has often led to a "practitioner mentality." Evidence that such is not a natural result of applied work can be seen with the applied anthropologists. Community training at a predoctoral level may best be represented in an introduction to the community and to field-research methods.

It is my view that the time has come for a review and perhaps a reconceptualization of applied psychology as a whole. This will define areas of common concern, overlapping function, and similarities in method and procedure. It might even lead to a common core of training for applied areas similar to the "core areas" of psychology adopted by many graduate departments of psychology.

In light of this view and the previous distinctions, one might view the process of becoming a professional psychologist as: first, education into the basics of general psychology; second, introduction to laboratory psychology; third, introduction to field psychology; fourth, specialization in laboratory or field methods with course work on basic or applied problems as indicated by the personal interest of the student. Community psychology would take its place as a field-research area with primary emphasis on applied problems.

REFERENCES

American Psychological Association (APA), Division of Counseling and Guidance, Committee on Counselor Training. Recommended standards for training counseling psychologists at the doctorate level. The practicum training of counseling psychologists. (Northwestern Conference) *Amer. Psychologist,* 1952, **7**, 175-188.

American Psychological Association (APA), Division of Community Psychology. *Newsletter,* Summer, 1966.

American Psychological Association (APA), Division of Community Psychology. *Newsletter,* June, 1967.

Barker, R. G. Roles, ecological niches, and the psychology of the absent organism. Paper presented at the Conference on the Propositional Structure of Role Theory, University of Missouri, March, 1962.

Bennett, C. C. , Anderson, Lurleen S., Cooper, S., Hassol, L., Klein, D. C., & Rosenblum, G. *Community psychology: a report of the Boston conference on the education of psychologists for community mental health,* May, 1965. Boston: Boston Univer. Press, 1966.

Bennis, W. G., Benne, K. D., & Chin, R. (Eds.) *The planning of change: readings in the applied behavioral sciences.* New York: Holt, Rinehart & Winston, 1961.

Berdie, R. F. Counseling principles and presuppositions. *J. counsel. Psychol.,* 1959, **6**, 175-182.

Bloom, B. L. The community mental health movement and the American social revolution. Paper presented at the Third Annual Professional Development Institute, Rocky Mountain Psychological Association, Albuquerque, New Mexico, May 11, 1966.

Bucher, R., & Strauss, A. Professions in process. *Amer. J. Sociol.,* 1960-1961, **66**, 325-334.

Duncan, O. D. Social organization and the ecosystem. In R. E. L. Faris (Ed.), *Handbook of modern sociology.* Chicago: Rand McNally, 1964.

Faris, R. E. L., & Dunham, H. W. *Mental disorders in urban areas: an ecological study of schizophrenia and other psychoses.* Chicago: Univer. of Chicago Press, 1939.

Fryer, D., & Henry, E. R. (Eds.) *Handbook of applied psychology.* New York: Rinehart, 1950. 2 vols.

Gouldner, A. W. Theoretical requirements of the applied social sciences. In W. G. Bennis, K. D. Benne, & R. Chin (Eds.), *The planning of change: readings in the applied behavioral sciences.* New York: Holt, Rinehart & Winston, 1961.

Hoch, E. L., Ross, A. O., & Winder, C. L. (Eds.) *Professional preparation of clinical psychologists.* Washington, D.C.: American Psychological Association, 1966.

Hunt, J. McV. Psychological services in the tactics of psychological science. *Amer. Psychologist,* 1952, **7**, 608-622.

Jacques, E. Social therapy: technocracy or collaboration. In W. G. Bennis, K. D. Benne, & R. Chin (Eds.), *The planning of change: readings in the applied behavioral sciences.* New York: Holt, Rinehart & Winston, 1961.

Kelly, J. G. The mental health agent in the urban community. Group for the Advancement of Psychiatry. *Symposium 10,* 1964, **55**, 474-494.

Klein, D. C. The Human Relations Service as a community mental health laboratory. Paper presented at the 25th Anniversary of the Psychiatry Service, Massachusetts General Hospital, Boston, October 15, 1960.

Knobel, M. Discussant's comments. In U.S. National Institute of Mental Health, *Community mental health:individual adjustment or social planning?* Washington, D.C.: National Clearinghouse for Mental Health Information, 1966.

Miller, J. G. Living systems: basic concepts. *Behav. Sci.,* 1965, **10,** 193-237.

Murphy, G. *Historical introduction to modern psychology.* (Rev. ed.) New York: Harcourt, Brace, 1949.

Newbrough, J. R. Clinical psychology: phoenix or dead-duck. In *Proc. of the conference on professional preparation of clinical psychologists.* Baltimore: Maryland State Department of Mental Hygiene, 1964.

Newbrough, J. R. Community mental health: a movement in search of a theory. In U.S. National Institute of Mental Health, *Community mental health: individual adjustment or social planning?* Washington, D.C.: National Clearinghouse for Mental Health Information, 1966. (a)

Newbrough, J. R. Community mental health: in pursuit of humanity. Paper presented at the Third Annual Professional Development Institute, Rocky Mountain Psychological Association, Albuquerque, New Mexico, May 11, 1966. (b)

Newbrough, J. R., Rhodes, W. C., & Seeman, J. The development of community psychology at George Peabody College. In I. Iscoe & C. Spielberger, *Community psychology: perspectives in training and research.* New York: Appleton-Century-Crofts, in press.

Pages, M. The sociotherapy of the enterprise. In W. G. Bennis, K. D. Benne, & R. Chin (Eds.), *The planning of change: readings in the applied behavioral sciences.* New York: Holt, Rinehart & Winston, 1961.

Paterson, D. G. Applied psychology comes of age. *J. consult. Psychol.,* 1940, **4,** 1-9.

Poffenberger, A. T. *Principles of applied psychology.* New York: Appleton-Century, 1942.

Raimy, V. C. (Ed.) *Training in clinical psychology.* New York: Prentice-Hall, 1950.

Rosen, G. Social stress and mental disease from the eighteenth century to the present: some origins of social psychiatry. *Milbank Memorial Fund Quart.,* 1959, **37,** 5-32.

Warren, R. L. *The community in America.* Chicago: Rand McNally, 1963.

CHAPTER 4

The Psychologist and Society: One Man's Adventure into Community Psychology

Howard E. Mitchell

Psychology has always represented to me a professional group with meaningful concern about the social issues facing our society. I have always found our professional colleagues responsive to debate, and finally ready to take action, on the social issues requiring immediate solution in our communities. The list of these issues appears to be increasing rather than decreasing as we live in a contemporary society which is in such a rapid state of transition. As a profession, we are concerned about the issues of war and peace, poverty, academic freedom, desegregation and discrimination, automation, and human rights versus property rights. Psychologists recognize the critical importance of attempting to distinguish the extent to which the relative effects of various factors—the increasing depersonalization of life, the lack of social function of adolescents, the erosion of moral values, the tensions resulting from racial discrimination, and the anxieties arising from nuclear hazard—are at the root of our manifest social frustrations.

Nevertheless, we have a tradition in psychology that has made us hesitant to be more directly involved in the "foxholes" of some of these social issues. Attention among professional psychologists has been recently focused upon issues of professionalization within psychology. I participated in the Conference on the Professional Preparation of Clinical Psychologists, organized by Division 12, in 1965, in which there was considerable discussion about the pressure being brought upon the APA to play a more forceful role in regard to the professional interests of psychology such as legislation, certification, insurance, and public relations.

TOWARD A DEFINITION OF
COMMUNITY PSYCHOLOGIST

As will become evident, I belong to a relatively small group of psychologists who have become directly involved in the mainstream of these social issues. Until receiving a preliminary draft of a report of the Boston Conference on the Education of Psychologists for Community Mental Health, I really did not know what kind of psychologist I was, in terms of most of my current activities. The small group which assembled at the Boston conference in May, 1965, made some attempt to define the scope of community psychology and the role of the community psychologist:

Intense, candid, and task oriented small group discussion at the beginning of the Conference led to a strongly expressed recognition that the participants were occupied not only with an interest in the community mental health movement, but more importantly, with a general sense that the time had come to expand psychology's area of inquiry and action. Participants referred to psychologists' participation in such diverse areas of national life as the Peace Corps, the anti-poverty effort, a broad movement into the field of education, and the development of the consultation function in an array of settings, as evidence of the fact that both knowledge about and competence in social change activities have developed in psychology over the past several decades (Bennett et al., 1966, p. 4).

Although the Boston conference was not ready to reach any consensus on a definition of community psychology and the role of the community psychologist, there was an attempt—with which I find myself at home:

The community psychologist should have the knowledge and skill to assess and modify the reciprocal relationships between individuals and the social systems with which they interact. He should utilize and integrate findings from psychology and the other social sciences which bear upon the individual-system variables. He must be acutely aware of the limitations of the current state of knowledge and art in the community psychology field and should therefore feel committed both to the generation of concepts and to the dissemination of knowledge in the field. The role of the community psychologist may therefore be seen as that of a "participant-conceptualizer." As such, he is clearly involved in and may be a mover of community processes, but he is also a professional attempting to conceptualize those processes within the framework of psychological-sociological knowledge (Bennett et al., 1966, pp. 7-8).

By such definition, I am a community psychologist. Like most of those so identified, I have moved into these areas from a primary training in and identification with mental health. I was basically trained as a clinical psychologist and the first half of my fifteen years of work was spent in clinical settings—initially in a Veterans Administration mental-hygiene clinic, a child-guidance clinic of a general medical hospital, and later in a social agency specializing in handling pre- and postmarital problems. It is my feeling that this clinical heritage provides a distinctive quality and concern when the psychologist becomes more engaged with man in his interface situation in the community.

I have started from the premise that psychology both as a science and as a profession is concerned with the basic social changes in society. These changes articulated by the civil-rights movement are so basic as to have been termed "revolutionary." I am assuming that psychology—as a science and as a profession— would be the last to want to play ostrich at times like these and bury its head in the cultural sands, hopeful upon emerging that things will be as they were. Thus, reflecting the feeling that learning is complete, the organism is satisfied, and society—indeed, the world—is in a state of equilibrium. No, my observations lead me to believe that both the scientific and the philosophical heritage of psychology make its disciples view the state-of-things with a healthy degree of skepticism. We are concerned about the social issues facing our contemporary society, although in only limited numbers are we professionally involved in the direction, planning, and research which are so essential. Essential because our scientific heritage and training makes us concerned about how best man should use his ideas and skills most effectively during this critical period of social change. The humanitarian qualities of psychologists, most forcibly appreciated by dint of their clinical training, made us aware of the results in terms of individual and collective human misery if individuals for whatever reason—mental or physical disease, constitutional inadequacy, racial, religious, or ethnic barriers—are denied the opportunity to realize their full potential. This can only take place in a society which promotes change by an orderly process.

The extent to which psychologists should be more directly engaged in such a process at various levels of decision making and planning, service, and research is the issue before us. The extent to which psychologists of all specialties are adequately trained for such ventures is another matter for consideration. The extent to which the organizational structure of psychology at local, state, and national levels is geared to be responsive to the social issues of our times is another matter.

I do not profess the wisdom nor the access of information to answer these questions. I invite you, however, to pursue the answers with me as I present a case history of my own involvement into the front lines of the "revolution" about us. By resorting to autobiographical data, I fully appreciate the risk I run with this audience. I shall expose both conscious and unconscious motivations to your analytical skills. Moreover, I also appreciate from our common clinical training how selective one should be in making personal references in clinical work. Nevertheless, what I have to say can best be said via a brief personal-professional excursion. What I will say reflects a professional life style which I feel has implications for psychology's response to society's problems.

ONE MAN'S ADVENTURE

The Early Years as Clinical Psychologist

Whatever I did during my initial years of work as a clinical psychologist in traditional roles of diagnostic and therapeutic work, I found the need to supplement these endeavors by involving myself in a variety of civic and public efforts. I served on boards of social agencies, health and welfare planning groups, the citizens' advisory group of the Philadelphia Housing Association, a child-guidance clinic, and an agency devoted to reducing intergroup tensions. Although I never saw my role as a psychologist nor sought to present the image of a psychologist, almost invariably my unique contribution to the various groups was as a professional psychologist. I found that I was welcomed as an active participant in the policy dialogue in the above organizations. My initial concern that such involvement would dissipate my scientific heritage or values was soon recognized mainly as a rationalization for not committing myself in unfamiliar territory. Moreover, I increasingly appreciated that the medical-clinical model was not appropriate for most of the complex issues being faced. Indeed, although in most of these complex social issues, it is still unclear what model is appropriate, at least one's social-scientific training makes one recognize the need for some frame of reference in order to discern the forest from the trees. As I have observed psychologists in these situations, they are able to analyze and specify the problems and recommend the means of intervention into the cultural setting in order to promote behavioral modification and social change.

Employment in a social agency, the Marriage Council of Philadelphia, which became a part of the University of Pennsylvania in 1952, opened new vistas. Concurrently, I served on the Committee on Relations with Social Work of the APA for two periods totaling six years at this time. The latter experience exposed me directly to the profession of social work and its traditional ways of community involvement. At this time in my own work, I moved toward research on clinical practice as I examined a variety of small-group problems in which I sought to bring social-psychological concepts to bear on clinical issues.

During my tenure as president of the Pennsylvania Psychological Association (1950-1960), I argued unsuccessfully for the association to lobby informally, along with social work and education, for child-welfare legislation then before the Commonwealth of Pennsylvania lawmakers. The energies and funds of the state association were absorbed in the immediate vested interest of establishing a program of self-certification. The attendance at both the state and local Philadelphia Society of Clinical Psychology was never as large at meetings on public or broad social issues as it was to discuss therapeutic techniques or clinical instruments. Perhaps this is all in the course of the history of organizational development. Personally, however, I began to lose interest and found these discussions as stale as most of the articles in psychological journals. They seemed for the most part to report imperceptible variations of old themes known for several decades.

Therefore in January, 1963, I accepted the opportunity to take a leave of absence from the University of Pennsylvania to become Associate Director of the Philadelphia Council for Community Advancement (PCCA). This organization was the fifth urban experiment then being conducted by the Ford Foundation to see if an "umbrella-type" structure could do something about the problems of the blighted areas of large urban communities. These organizational structures were the prototypes of the community-action groups in large urban areas under the war-on-poverty programs. The PCCA, like many such community-action organizations in the current poverty campaign, was literally pulled apart by external and internal power struggles. There was little opportunity systematically to design and carry out programs. However, this learning experience was invaluable in terms of the challenging opportunity which followed.

We hear much today about exciting new roles and opportunities for social scientists and psychologists in community mental-health facilities and in training the nonprofessional and the subprofessional. Most of this work is related to mental-health programs and facilities. My emerging role as a community psychologist since April, 1964, has been, however, in working from the base of a large urban university. It is from this point of vantage that I want to talk about how I have become engaged in the social issues facing one large metropolis.

The Role of the University

The universities of America have been busily engaged in initiating programs whose aim it is to help every citizen more fully utilize his potential in our society. This is a role which I feel the large urban university can play most effectively—a role which I feel the University of Pennsylvania by action of enlightened, sensitive leadership of its president is playing. We have come to realize that our colleges and universities are embedded in our culture and our society and that fundamental or widespread change in these institutions can come about only when there is a shift of emphasis in our general system of values or when there is a change in our general societal processes. At the same time, however, the direction of my influence may be the other way; there is an *interaction* of the college or university on the one hand, and the surrounding society and culture on the other.

Our society is now looking to its schools and colleges—expectantly, urgently—as the principal agency to make the dream of democracy come true, to assure freedom of opportunity to every boy and girl, no matter how forbidding and difficult the school or family circumstances may be. The country is aroused and interested in the problems of equalizing opportunity, and Americans are persuaded of the great power of education. Many colleges and universities have responded.

The institutions of higher education are occupied as never before with the complex and important work in developing programs of all sorts for disadvantaged youth. This work involves new approaches in the recruitment of talented youngsters of low-income groups, changes in the manner in which financial aid is given to needy students, and a close look at admission policies and the degree to which assessment techniques are culturally biased. Recently, some universities have recognized that they must identify the talented student much before the twelfth-grade level if he is to be readied to compete in schools of higher learning. Partnerships between white and Negro universities and colleges have recently developed, which include programs of student and faculty exchange and cultural programs and curricular experimentation and advice.

[Between October 1963 and 1965 alone], the major educational foundations ... invested nearly $40 million in grants designed to further the cause of expanding educational opportunities in the nation's colleges and universities. This new level of financial support reflects not only the heightened interest of the major foundations in stimulating "opportunity for equality", but also the renewed sense of dedication and concern that has marked developments in this field on campuses in all parts of the country (American Council of Education, 1965).

An Example: The University of Pennsylvania

It has been the policy of the University of Pennsylvania, under President Gaylord P. Harnwell, to react with sensitivity to the important and pressing problems that relate to the equality of opportunity for all American citizens in their communal life. The university has been viewed as having an important and appropriate role to play in community evolution and in stimulating the fair and impartial development of the nation's and the community's human resources. This role is perceived as one requiring a rational approach, thoughtful concern, and the studied employment of the best policies and practices that present understanding of complex human relationships permit.

The university has been engaged in the development of a geographical sector of West Philadelphia (where the university is located) in the creation of a "university city." This project has involved integrating the expanding educational institution with the total life of the surrounding community. The West Philadelphia Corporation was established to revitalize the community in all of its central dimensions—educational, recreational, housing, health, and other community services. Under dynamic leadership, the West Philadelphia Corporation has sparked imaginative programs and has established itself as a sound medium of university-community interaction.

Students at the university, like students around the world, are in the vanguard of freedom. In early 1964, one student-leadership group at the university presented the president with a nine-point action program concerning the hiring practices and apprenticeship policies of the building and construction trades engaged in raising new structures on the campus. In response to this inquiry, it was publicly announced that the university does have a responsibility—a genuine desire—actively to support equality of opportunity. With members of the student protest group in attendance, meetings were held with representatives of all building and construction contractors engaged in university work. President Harnwell made it eminently clear in these discussions that the university was committed to the democratic ideal and considered the antidiscrimination clause to be a vital part of every contract with them.

These discussions also made clear the opportunity for students, faculty, and administration to have a meaningful impact upon the life of people in the community, as well as an opportunity for students, faculty, and administration to widen their horizons and experience. Much consideration was given to the most effective instrument to accomplish these objectives. Attention was given by the university administration as to the most effective administrative mechanism which would immediately bring the resources of the university to bear upon the "urban condition." Moreover, this entity should operate within keeping the university's primary function of adding to knowledge and training.

The Human Resources Program

In April, 1964, the Human Resources Program was established at the university by President Harnwell as a broad thrust to develop the usefulness of underemployed elements of society. This program was charged with the responsibility of *coordinating student, faculty, and administrative efforts in the areas of education, human and industrial relations with special reference to social change and equality of opportunity.* As program director, I was made responsible to the Office of the President. Policy is enunciated by a Human Resources Council, drawn from several faculties of the university and headed by Dean Jefferson B. Fordham of the law school.

The first major project of the Human Resources Program was a six-week summer educational and vocational program and follow-up study of 100 male unemployed high-school dropouts from the Philadelphia area. Financed by a grant from the United States Office of Education, it was a pilot project for the Urban Job Corps Training Centers then envisioned by the Economic Opportunity Act of 1964, and currently in operation across the country. We sought to develop guidelines for these larger projects, exploring how best to recruit out-of-school, unemployed youth, the limitations of assessment techniques, the initial engagements between middle-income VISTA type resident counselors and the low-income students, the test of experimental education techniques and reward systems, and the extent to which self-government could be effective in these residential programs.

The trainees, of whom 67 were Negro and 33 white, lived in university dormitories during each week and went home weekends. They spent mornings in remedial reading, mathematics, and communication-skills classes. In the afternoons, they were assigned to vocational projects in the community or in university departments, for which they were paid $10 per week and an additional $25 upon completion of the program.

Evenings were devoted to recreational and cultural activities, including basketball games, jam sessions, "town meetings," and a trip to a summer theater. A student governing council, elected by the trainees, gave them a voice in planning their own activities as well as experience in leadership and group participation.

Of the original 100 trainees, 90 completed the program. The follow-up study conducted within three months after the end of the project revealed that about 60 per cent had obtained one or more jobs, 30 per cent had returned to school, and 10 per cent had gotten into difficulty with the law. However, a sizable number of those who obtained jobs requiring little skill, substandard pay and working conditions were already back on urban streetcorners, eager to be involved in more extended residential vocational programs.

This pilot project enabled social scientists, psychologists, and educators to study and measure students' reactions to various educational innovations and motivational procedures. Interestingly, although we had great need for psychological personnel, the few who were contacted rejected our invitations. By contrast, sociology, planning, and education students were eager to be a part of this program.

Another project sponsored by the Human Resources Program was a 13-week televised course in Negro history and culture, carried by two Philadelphia stations. The course could be taken for credit in the university's College of General Studies or viewed simply as an informative television series. The course dealt with the historical, social, and cultural factors contributing to the suppression of the Negro in American society, the variety of response to his plight, and his attempts to improve his circumstances through the means available to him. Half-hour lectures were given three times a week by university professors and 15 guest authorities. The lectures were taped by the Commonwealth of Pennsylvania for use in state-supported teacher-training institutions. A small foundation grant was obtained so that the research staff of the Human Resources Program could evaluate the effectiveness of this course.

To prepare teachers for the challenges of the inner-city school, the Human Resources Program organized and offered a course, in the spring of 1963, entitled "Education in Large Urban Areas," for students in the University of Pennsylvania's graduate teacher-intern program. The course focuses on factors affecting education in major cities and gives special attention to the culturally disadvantaged child—to the development of personality in what Nevitt Sanford (1966) calls "the change-producing institutions of society."

During the summer of 1965, two additional projects were carried out. In cooperation with Plans for Progress[1] and the school district of Philadelphia, a three-week institute was held for the purpose of increasing the professional competence of high-school guidance counselors in their work with students of low-income family situations. Two follow-up workshops were held with this group in which special projects designed during the institute were critiqued. These projects covered a wide range of individual and

[1]Plans for Progress is comprised of business and industrial firms who have pledged themselves to support the President's Committee on Equal Job Opportunity.

group counseling techniques and the measurement of their effectiveness.

The other program initiated in June, 1965, provided a transitional experience for 50 high-school youngsters of low-income background, who had been accepted for college in the fall of 1965 but had specific remedial needs. The intent was to better ready them for their forthcoming matriculation in universities of higher learning by involving them in a process whereby they were exposed to a greater choice of activities and counseled in regard to the consequences of their behavior in this new situation. Crucial issues before many of the colleges and universities which are actively seeking "culturally disadvantaged" youth who have the potential to successfully negotiate their programs are (1) how to identify such individuals, and (2) how to provide them with the type of environment which will enable them to complete the academic experience in greater numbers.

In keeping with that part of the charge to the Human Resources Program to coordinate student activities, we are currently engaged in making known to our student body all off-campus undergraduate service opportunities in metropolitan Philadelphia. This work is largely the product of an undergraduate committee to which the Human Resources Program provides appropriate staff and technical assistance.

Time does not permit even citing other programs being developed by the Human Resources Program. All of the programs that have been carried out or are on the drawing board encompass a wide range of our knowledge about human behavior. Moreover, working from the base of an urban university, I find myself directly immersed in the challenging problems facing our society—antipoverty efforts, the training of teachers of the "culturally disadvantaged," the training of the nonprofessional, and how to make the young college student's search for identity through his involvement with social-change processes more meaningful.

In its first two years, the Human Resources Program designed and carried out experimental programs dealing with a wide range of urban problems. The internal and external impact of these experiments illuminated both the academic opportunities and the public responsibilities inherent in the university's situation. Cognizant of its opportunities and responsibilities, the University of Pennsylvania, in the spring of 1966, took a series of steps looking toward the growth and permanence of the Human Resources Program:

1. The Human Resources Program, as an action-research agency, became part of the Institute for Environmental Studies, the research arm of the university's Departments of Architecture, City Planning, and Landscape Architecture and Regional Planning.

2. A university Council on Urbanism and Human Resources was formed (replacing the former "advisory committee" to the Human Resources Program) and directed to consider the establishment of a Department of Urbanism and Human Resources in the Graduate School of Arts and Sciences.

3. As Director of the Human Resources Program, I was appointed Professor of Human Resources in the Department of City and Regional Planning. By action of the Trustees of the University of Pennsylvania in October, 1967, the 1907 Foundation Professorship in Urbanism and Human Resources was established and I was appointed the first incumbent to this chair.

Within the Department of City and Regional Planning, the Human Resources Program has been involved in developing the social-planning curriculum; assisting in introductory courses taken by students of planning, civic design, and architecture; participating in planning juries; coordinating community-based field studies; and research and counseling to private and public agencies on the human aspects of urbanism.

A course entitled "Urban Social Change and Human Development" was designed to assist the planning student in understanding the process of social change in the urban environment through studying the attitudes of low-income and minority populations toward housing, urban renewal, education, employment, and welfare services. The course emphasizes both the need for planning institutions to render human services more effectively and the development of a conceptual framework for comprehensive planning.

A special readings seminar has also been developed to familiarize the planning student with interdisciplinary literature on poverty, combined with intensive field experiences in a critical slum area near the university. From these teaching and action-research functions, a comprehensive model is being developed for urban slum renewal strategy.

Looking toward the future, it is the mission of the Human Resources Program to increase our knowledge about the human aspects of urbanism, to provide the best professional training, and to develop new approaches. More effective planning methods, which include greater emphasis upon human and social factors, are continually being investigated. To strengthen the social-physical planning curriculum, priority will be given to action-research and training in the following areas:

1. Undergraduate and graduate instruction in urbanism and human resources.

2. Social-engineering aspects of planning to provide better-coordinated human resources in the urban complex.

3. Community development and training issues.

4. Urban intervention strategies, including the organizational framework of the urban slum—its power network and communications system.

CONCLUSION: PSYCHOLOGISTS AND THE COMMUNITY

In the preface to his book, Sam Bass Warner has a statement which I find points up why psychologists are needed in the planning sciences.

In a democratic society, the goal of planning is not to promote one particular style of urban living; rather, the goal of planning is to create humane environments which will widen the choices open to individual city dwellers and will enrich the many cultural styles that now exist. Current American urban environments considerably restrict individual choice, and they foster a good deal of self-distinctive behavior in all cultural styles (Warner, 1966).

The individualizing of man's behavior has always been an area in which psychologists have made a significant contribution.

There is a great need for larger numbers of psychologists to be trained to join in these efforts. It seems to me that psychology has an opportunity as never before to bring its skills to bear on some of the issues facing our communities. Already the promise of psychology's contribution is great, as one looks at Jerome Bruner's innovative work in education, Nicholas Hobb's approach to mental retardation and child development, and the efforts of Nevitt Sanford and his associates in the field of alcoholism at the Institute for the Study of Human Problems, Stanford University.

All of the above pioneering work has brought these psychologists into a more direct interface with man in his natural habitat. This is where many of the problems are, which require our skills. Not only can society ill afford not to utilize the talents of the profession of psychology, but every psychologist who has become so involved reports feeling richer personally and professionally.

REFERENCES

American Council of Education. *Expanding opportunities: the Negro and higher education*, Vol. II, No. 1, January, 1965.

Bennett, C. C., Anderson, Lurleen S., Cooper, S., Hassol, L., Klein, D. C., & Rosenblum, G. *Community psychology: a report of the Boston conference on the education of psychologists for community mental health*, May, 1965. Boston: Boston Univer. Press, 1966.

Sanford, N. *Self and society: social change and individual development.* New York: Atherton Press, 1966.

Warner, S. B., Jr. (Ed.) *Planning for a nation of cities.* Cambridge: M.I.T. Press, 1966.

II

TOWARD
A THEORETICAL
FRAMEWORK

The theoretical chapters included in Part II address three central aspects of the contribution from community psychology to conceptualization:

1. What does the field demand in the way of novel theoretical constructs, and does community mental health have special conceptual requirements?
2. What can familiar concepts contribute to our understanding, and what modifications of traditional theory are occurring?
3. What are the implications of both new and old theories for research and action?

Crisis theory is most frequently associated with the community mental-health field as a relatively new conceptual model. In Chapter 5, Kalis evaluates the present status of this theory and charts some directions for its development. She examines the relationships of crisis theory to stress theories and disaster theories, the similarities and differences between concepts of accidental crises and developmental crises, and the enrichment that crisis theory can provide to the understanding of ecologies and the planning of preventive intervention.

The contributions of role theory and the structure of social identity to the understanding of the community psychologist's function as change agent are elaborated by Sarbin in Chapter 6. He underlines, as do a number of authors throughout this volume, the necessity of considering ecological variables in all community conceptualizations. In Sarbin's view, the objectives of community psychology differ from those of psychologists in other settings, and he details the ways in which he considers the metaphors of role theory to be appropriate, and those of other theoretical constructs to be inappropriate, for the attainment of these different objectives.

Adelson's chapter, which follows, develops a framework around the concepts of self-valuation, social valuation, and self-identity as an explanatory approach to the problem of growth and adaptation. He illustrates the meaningfulness of such a theoretical framework in relation to a variety of behavior disorders, for the understanding of minority-group actions in their search for identity and for research and practice implications in social and community psychology.

In the next chapter, Kelly invokes principles from field biology as a basis for developing research on social environments. In distinction to the more familiar employment of sociological or cultural concepts of ecology, this author attempts to avoid a purely descriptive psychological ecology and demonstrates the translation of biological principles to community-psychology concerns. He summarizes his study of adaptive behavior in varied high-school environments as an illustration of the cogency of his conceptualizations. Thus, this chapter is a bridge, as is Chapter 9, by Nevitt Sanford, to Part III on research and action.

In his discussion of community actions for the prevention of alcoholism, Sanford points out that the interdisciplinary nature of work on the alcoholism problem can be generalized to the whole of the community mental-health field. He gives careful attention to definitional considerations in preventive intervention and contributes to the consensus that contextual variables and wide-range conceptualization and intervention are inescapable features of community psychology. In a detailed discussion of a typology of alcohol problems and their interrelationships and approaches to prevention, he illustrates these principles by developing a plan which includes changes in the law and changes in institutional settings (schools) and which is theoretically based on well-documented psychodynamic considerations.

Each of the five authors in this part presents a somewhat different perspective on the status of theory building in community psychology and community mental health. But they agree on the necessity of including considerations of context, of ecology, or of man in his environment. They also clearly refute any impression that the field is developing without any theoretical base. While several references are made to the conceptual contributions from other disciplines, it is apparent that community psychologists are, in a major way, concerned with the evolution of theory for the community mental-health field.

CHAPTER 5

Crisis Theory: Its Relevance for Community Psychology and Directions for Development

Betty L. Kalis

As the field of community psychology develops, a number of conceptual models are appropriately being invoked in understanding and guiding research and practice. Concepts of crisis and crisis intervention appear with increasing frequency in the literature and seem to have particular cogency for community mental health. This chapter outlines the areas of consensus about crisis theory and analyzes the present status of theoretical development, using a paradigm suggested by Chapman (1962) for analyzing theoretical approaches to disaster.

AREAS OF CONSENSUS AND DIVERGENCE

Most traditional psychological theories focus on intrapersonal and interpersonal variables as the crucial predictors of behavior. Concern with community problems has led to the recognition that more explicitly ecological considerations need to be taken into account, and crisis theory can be categorized as one of several ecological theories from which meaningful hypotheses and predictions can be generated and tested. The general concern of ecology is with the mutual relations between organisms and their environment. Some theories tend to focus primarily on the impact of environments upon people, to the conceptual neglect of the "mutuality" in the definition. Others center on adaptive tasks and alloplastic capacities of person-members of the ecology, and give less attention to environmental variables. Crisis theory is concerned with those phenomena which Deevey (1963) has characterized as ecological "wobble," and attempts to elucidate the interdependent nature of organismic and environmental variables.

While all ecological theories share some common assumptions, it is useful to recognize that crisis theory falls conceptually between stress theories and disaster theories and incorporates concepts from each. Stress theories, as exemplified by the careful research of Janis (1958), principally approach the understanding of personality characteristics and coping devices which are predictive of adaptation to an external stressor. (Janis's major work has related to planned surgery.) Control is directed toward altering the state of the individual through anticipatory guidance so as to effect a more favorable adaptive prognosis. The theory and research pertaining to naturally occurring life stress are most directly related to crisis theory. Theoretical refinement is occurring, however, out of laboratory stress research, such as that of Lazarus (1966) and others.

Disaster theories, on the other hand, have usually approached the understanding of behavior in the face of catastrophe based on an analysis of features of the disastrous events. Thus, the systematic definition of a disastrous event proposed by Marks and Fritz (1954) and the framework of disaster stages outlined by Powell et al. (1953) to permit comparisons between disasters are both community-oriented and concerned with the impact of environmental events.

This perhaps exaggerated distinction between the two kinds of theories draws attention to a theoretical dilemma: Even when the problem under investigation is clearly ecological, variables important for one aspect of understanding are different from those for another, and bridging concepts and interaction variables are not ordinarily a part of a single theoretical system. Although crisis theory, in its present stage of development, attempts to bridge this gap, specific constructs for doing so are in a rudimentary stage, as will be apparent from the remainder of the chapter.

The diversity of definitions and the lack of clarity about even the concept of crisis have been commented on by a number of writers. Lydia Rapoport differentiates between concepts of accidental and developmental crises, and limits consideration to the former in community mental health. She cites Caplan's (1963) broad definition of crisis as an "upset in a steady state" and lists three sets of interrelated factors which can produce a state of crisis: "(1) a hazardous event which poses some threat; (2) a threat to instinctual need which is symbolically linked to earlier threats that resulted in vulnerability or conflict; and (3) an inability to respond with adequate coping mechanisms" (Rapoport, 1962, p. 213).

Miller and Iscoe (1963) found consensus that crises are time-limited, associated with changed behavior which may lead to unfavorable outcome, and characterized by feelings of helplessness and tension which find varied expression. While their review of the literature emphasized the idiosyncratic nature of perceived threat leading to crisis, more recently Jacobson et al. (1968) made a useful distinction between such individual crises and what they call generic crises which can be predicted for population groups.

Elsewhere (1966) the author has suggested that since both organismic and environmental factors are part of the definition of crisis, a useful concept would be a continuum with respect to the origins of crisis, ranging from those crises precipitated primarily by a hazardous environmental event to those primarily originating out of personal vulnerability. Such a framework might clarify the definitional problems encountered by judges in Bloom's (1963) study, who could not identify the crisis state without knowledge of a precipitating stress. A similar continuum would be relevant regarding the locus of crisis intervention, with environmental manipulation at one pole and intervention in intrapsychic processes at the other. These suggestions elaborate the theoretical underpinnings of crisis in indicating that

1. The disruption of equilibrium characteristic of the crisis state is independent of the origin of the disruption.
2. The intervention leading to the resolution of crisis and the restoration of equilibrium is independent both of the disruption and of its origin.

Schulberg and Sheldon (1968) propose a probabilistic formulation of crisis which takes into account the probability that a hazardous event will occur, the probability that an individual will be exposed to this event, and the vulnerability of the individual to the event. They indicate that such a formulation can lead not only to predictions of crises but also to alternative strategies for preventive intervention.

PRESENT STATUS OF CRISIS THEORY: NINE DIMENSIONS

This outline of definitional consensus and diversity has been presented as an introduction to the analysis of the present status of crisis theory and the usefulness of its concepts in relation to various kinds of community mental-health problems. Chapman (1962) suggests that nine dimensions can be employed to examine the properties of theoretical models:

1. *Implication*
   Descriptive (and hollow) ←——————→ Implicated (and filled)
2. *Situational Reference*
   Individual ←——————————————————→ Situational
3. *Level of Abstraction*
   Low-Level ←——————————————————→ High-Level
4. *Systematic Unity*
   Eclectic ←————————————————→ Systematically Unified
5. *Comprehensiveness*
   Segmental ←————————————————→ Comprehensive
6. *Temporal Extension*
   Contemporary-Field ←————————→ Time-Extended
7. *Spatial Extension*
   Local ←————————————————————→ Space-Extended
8. *Manipulability of Variables*
   Nonmanipulable ←————————————→ Manipulable
9. *Evolutionism*
   Static ←————————————————————→ Developmental

While this paradigm was developed for the analysis of disaster theories, it lends itself as well to exploring the ramifications of crisis theory.

1. IMPLICATION

This dimension concerns the development of laws and regularities which govern the variables covered by the model, how far it has proceeded from description to a fully elaborated set of constructs and intervening variables which account for the relationships between input and output. Despite the proliferation of crisis-theory literature as reflected in bibliographies such as the one prepared by Rochman (1965), crisis theory is clearly in its infancy and remains largely at the descriptive end of the continuum. Refinement of concepts and definitions, and problems of generalization across studies, are the main arenas of theoretical development to date. In view of community mental-health concerns with populations and not only with individuals, three general kinds of predictive indices are needed:

1. What kinds of events can be predicted to evoke crises in large numbers of persons?

2. What kinds of populations-at-risk can be identified, by reason of special vulnerability, in relation to events?

3. What kinds of interventions are specific for the favorable resolution of what kinds of crises?

Even though these questions have not been settled, crisis theory has moved toward implication with a set of consensual assumptions:

1. That human functioning requires the maintenance of an ongoing homeostasis or equilibrium not only within the organism but in relationship to the environment.

2. That any disruption of this equilibrium is followed by attempts to restore it or to achieve a new adaptive balance.

3. That certain disruptive periods can, by their characteristics, be identified as crisis states.

4. That behaving organisms are more susceptible to external influence during a period of disruption than during a period of stable equilibrium.

5. That the period of disruption is self-limited and may be followed by a new adaptation which is qualitatively different from the one which preceded the disruption.

6. That equilibrium can be restored by changing features of the environment, changing modes of coping, or both.

These assumptions are serving as guiding principles for both research and crisis intervention; and with continuing feedback from these sources, the model probably will move closer to the implicative end of the continuum.

2. SITUATIONAL REFERENCE

This is a dimension which ranges from the social and physical situation at one end to the individual within these situations at the other. The literature on crisis details both the properties of events probabilistically predictive of crisis evocation and the nature of adaptive and maladaptive behavior syndromes for individuals in crisis states. Interaction variables are considerably less well explicated at this point in time.

With respect to events, the sources are scattered, but it is possible to spell out some kinds of event properties which combine probabilistically to predict high-risk groups for experiencing crisis. Many of the variables have emerged from the exceedingly detailed research on disaster, which may be conceptualized as crisis at the extreme environmental end of the origins-of-crisis continuum. The predictors have some generality for individual crises as well. Included would be factors such as suddenness, magnitude, duration, intensity, and proximity.

Two interaction concepts, between event and vulnerability, are (1) degree of control over the occurrence of the event and (2) frequency. To illustrate the importance of the control factor, research on the crisis of relocation such as that reported by Fried (1963) has amply documented the increased crisis potential of an imposed move as distinguished from one that is actively sought. When frequency versus uniqueness is viewed as a bridge or interaction concept, it is necessary to consider both the carryover of learning or mastery from one crisis to another and the presence or absence of community supports for dealing with repetitive events with high risk properties. A worker's ability to cope with periodic losses of employment may depend upon his self-esteem, his flexibility in changing roles, and his capacity to prepare for times without an income. At the community level, however, these factors need to be matched by the presence of alternative employment opportunities, training programs for persons whose skills are rendered obsolete by technological advances, and so on.

Thus, the potential for crisis can be conceptually delineated both in terms of what people can do as a function of their own learning, adaptability, flexibility, and personal competence to deal with the inevitable changes and vicissitudes of life, and in terms of what a community needs to provide in relation to hazardous events, independent of its inhabitants' internal resources and capacity to cope. If it is assumed that successful mastery of crises can constitute important growth experiences, since meaningful changes in adaptive patterns can emerge from disruptions of equilibrium, then community planners must consider what supports can be built in at a community-wide level to promote such successful mastery.

One reason for the saliency of crisis concepts in community-psychology literature is this opportunity and growth-potential aspect, the focus on competence and on coping. While it is essential to remain aware of the dangerous features inherent in the crisis state, to the extent that planning and intervention are in the area of facilitating adaptive coping with crisis, it is a conceptual model which focuses away from the more traditional clinical concern with psychopathology.

At the same time, in order to facilitate adaptive coping, knowledge of adaptive and maladaptive patterns of response is necessary. Some of the richest research findings are in this area, beginning with Lindemann's (1944) studies of acute grief and bereavement, and Bowlby's (1952) observations on reactions to mother-child separation. Since those relatively early studies, knowledge of a number of other common situational and accidental crises has developed (see Parad, 1965).

The kinds of characteristics which cut across different crises and reflect effective and ineffective patterns of coping have been conceptualized in several different ways. They have been summarized by Caplan (1963), who suggests that adaptive coping requires:

1. Active exploration of reality issues and search for information.

2. Free expression of both positive and negative feelings and a tolerance of frustration.

3. Active invoking of help from others.

4. Breaking problems down into manageable bits and working through them one at a time.

5. Awareness of fatigue and tendencies toward disorganization, with pacing of efforts and maintenance of control in as many areas of functioning as possible.

6. Active mastery of feelings where possible, and acceptance of inevitability where not. Flexibility and willingness to change.

7. Basic trust in themselves and others and basic optimism about outcome.

Maladaptive coping, on the other hand, is characterized by:

1. Avoidance or denial of problems with judgments based upon

wish-fulfillment or fantasy rather than reality.

2. Avoidance and denial of negative feelings; dealing with them by projection or blaming when they do break through.

3. When denial and avoidance break down, massive and generalized disorganization of functioning involving most areas of living.

4. Inability to pace themselves; either overactivity or underactivity.

5. Inability to seek or accept help from others.

6. Reacting globally or stereotypically to problems; feeling easily overwhelmed.

There is general theoretical agreement, then, on the importance of both intrapsychic and environmental factors in the initiation and termination of disruptive individual crisis states. Intervention at preventive and control levels, however, is more often a function of the character of the intervening force than it is the demands of the situation per se. That is, for example, the psychotherapist has attended for the most part to the intrapsychic and interpersonal phenomena; the attention of agents of social change, on the other hand, has centered on the complex of environmental forces. The domain of community mental health affords an opportunity to coalesce these two approaches.

In individual crises the chief concern is often with intrapsychic variables and the immediate life space of the individual. In those papers which report on family crises, an interesting conceptual shift occurs as the social system is expanded to encompass the family. Not only do the central variables change from intrapersonal to interpersonal, but it is the dynamic equilibrium of the family as a social system that becomes disrupted in the crisis state. In this new perspective, interventions are external to the individual although they may be internal to the family. Hill (1958) has explicated this point in detail.

Thus, the intervention alternatives in relation to an individual in crisis are different from those for a family in crisis, although resolution of crisis for either requires attention to factors within the system as well as those impinging upon it from without. In practice, the professional working with an individual assumes that resolution of the crisis state for that individual will facilitate the reestablishment of family equilibrium. Another alternative for the family, which the professional working at that level might support, would be to reestablish an equilibrium by extruding the individual. Some of the consequences of this conceptual differentiation for community mental health are illustrated in a study by Mercer (1966). She demonstrated that the probability of a family's reaccepting a retarded family member could be predicted from the knowledge of the crisis that led to institutionalization.

The extrapolations from this point have major relevance for community psychology, because one complication of conceptualization is that the object of study and attention is extremely variable. In relation to a given problem, concern may successively involve an individual, a family, a population at risk, a community agency or institution, or a community as a whole as variously defined. Both the disruption of equilibrium and the intervention at any point in any system have implications and reverberations at all levels and for all interlocking systems. Effective intervention, therefore, requires an awareness of the context in which intervention is being contemplated and of the various social systems, from individual to community, which are involved.

An important area of preventive intervention is that of mitigating the crisis potential of planned community change, such as changing the racial balance of schools, redevelopment and relocation, and the like. Even though the disruptive force is clear and the environmental change a "given" in such potential crises, appropriate interventions will vary from individual to individual, from family to family, among various ethnic and socioeconomic groups, and from community to community in relation to available resources and alternatives.

To summarize to this point, filling-in of the crisis model is proceeding with respect to both event properties and adaptive patterns. While there is recognition of the importance of interaction variables, specific research in this area is minimal. Studies of environment tend to be community-oriented or population-oriented, and studies of adaptive patterns tend to be individual-oriented or family-oriented. A comment of Chapman's regarding disaster research is highly applicable here:

At the time of the first serious research on disaster we had very good models of the physical nature of the disaster engendering forces and we had considerable psychological knowledge about the reaction of individuals to particular features in their social situation. This situation leads one to hope for a third model intervening between these two. This must be a model of the social situation induced by the output of the physical model which in turn has stimulus effects upon the individual such that his behavior can be understood as a function of that social situation (Chapman, 1962, p. 310).

3. LEVEL OF ABSTRACTION

Chapman describes this dimension as varying from extreme generality to extreme specificity of terms and relations. As theories and models reach higher and higher levels of abstraction, they tend to become less discriminate with respect to empirical problems.

Crisis theory is particularly oriented to behavior during change or flux, as distinguished from an interest in predicting the ongoing, steady state. Its field-dependent character, described under Dimension 6, Temporal Extension, also keeps it close to the specific pole of the Level of Abstraction continuum. While many of its constructs involve the interrelationships between environment and behavior, its problems of ecology are not the ones which have occupied ecological investigators such as Barker (1965) and Kelly (Chap. 8 of this volume). These theorists are interested in the differential prediction of behavior as a function of different persons in different environments. Crisis theory, on the other hand, focuses on behavioral changes which occur concomitantly with environmental changes, so that while the two interests are complementary, they are not identical. Both kinds of theorists share a preference for naturalistic settings as opposed to simulated environments or laboratory research. Naturalistic observations require the consideration of multiple variables, thus increasing the specificity of the resultant theoretical constructs.

4. SYSTEMATIC UNITY

A model may be highly systematic, with integrated variables, or it may contain a number of submodels, each explaining a different aspect of the whole.

Crisis theory clearly falls on the latter end of this dimension, as is apparent from the discussion under Situational Reference. Variables relating to events are largely borrowed from various disaster studies and are in a different class from variables used to explain coping and adaptation. Intrapersonal variables are largely derived from stress research and psychoanalytic theories of ego functioning. The primitive interaction variables which have been tested are only beginning to unify these submodels. A test of the predictive value of an interaction variable might require a comparative community study. To cite another example from the area of relocation and redevelopment, communities differ in the extent of resident participation during the planning phase of redevelopment. If personal control over the occurrence of a hazardous event is a predictive interaction variable, there should be fewer relocation-engendered crises in a participative community than in a nonparticipative one.

Moreover, since crisis theory fits into a broad ecological framework, the phenomena with which it is concerned require for their understanding variables from sociology, anthropology, and other social sciences as well as from other psychological theories. Specific vulnerability to certain hazardous events may be related to social class, the values of an ethnic minority, the political power structure, or the economic base of a community. Collaborative research which addresses these aspects of vulnerability can lead to the identification of high-risk groups, delineation of needs for community supports, and other data which are crucial for crisis prevention and intervention.

5. COMPREHENSIVENESS

This dimension assesses whether the theory explains the total range of phenomena under consideration or some restricted part of them. The eclecticism described above is a function of the attempt at comprehensiveness, but the potential for comprehensiveness is not yet fully developed. In community mental-health practice, crisis-oriented clinics—such as those described by Kalis et al. (1961), Hirsh (1960), Jacobson et al. (1965), and many others —have contributed to the understanding of individual crisis states and their resolution. Crisis and noncrisis reactions to hazardous events—described by Janis (1958), Kaplan and Mason (1960), Bibring et al. (1961), and others—have enhanced knowledge about vulnerability and coping styles. Janis (1958), Caplan (1964), and others have reported on the use of anticipatory guidance to avert crises, and Mayo and Klein (1964) have outlined some criteria for assessing the area of greatest disequilibrium among community subsystems.

These developments indicate that a crisis framework is useful

for understanding all phases of preventive intervention, for guiding community planning and development, and for conceptualizing process in mental-health consultation. Expansion of the model
to maximize this usefulness requires more multidisciplinary collaboration and integration of research findings than has yet occurred. Segmental aspects of crisis, therefore, are at present more
fully elaborated theoretically than is the total phenomenon.

6. TEMPORAL EXTENSION

This dimension refers not only to the total time embraced by the
model but also to the time dimension in relation to the pattern of
causes which are related to output. It is a very important dimension for this analysis, since crisis theory is relatively field-dependent and ahistorical in nature, with historical features considered
only as they are reactivated by and relevant to current crises.

The principal focus of the theory is on behavior in time of crisis,
usually defined as between a few days and about six weeks. Although this analysis is confined to concepts of accidental crisis, the
need for rapprochement with theories of developmental crises is
elucidated under Dimension 9, Evolutionism.

The crisis research concerned with the anticipatory-guidance
dimension, the opportunity to prepare for unavoidable hazardous
events, is aimed at averting crises and facilitating adaptive coping.
The extension of research interest to an anticipatory phase does
not, however, modify the time-limited conception of the crisis
state.

Silverman (1967) has commented on evidence of the working-
through of the mourning process in widows long after the presumed resolution of the crisis state following bereavement.
Current conceptualization would regard these "residuals" as part
of the adaptive pattern in the new equilibrium, but they clearly
have implications for the assessment of vulnerability to new crises.
These findings may stimulate interest in other follow-up studies
and in the assessment of differences between precrisis equilibrium
and a new adaptive balance. For the most part, however, crisis
research by definition deals with a clearly truncated time unit.

7. SPATIAL EXTENSION

This dimension is more easily understood in relation to disaster
theories than to crisis theory. Spatial extension would be charac-

terized by a model which considered the utmost spatial geographic limits within which can be found events relevant to the disaster or to products of it, as distinguished from models restricted to events having an immediate relationship to behavior.

With respect to crisis theory, this dimension can be translated in two ways which may help to dissipate some conceptual confusion. In the first instance, it may be taken to refer to the *magnitude* of hazardous events appropriate to the definition of crisis. At the extended pole, the question arises as to whether disaster should continue to be considered a special instance of crisis or whether it has enough distinctive aspects to warrant complete conceptual separation. At the individual pole, on the other hand, it may be asserted that personalized, as distinguished from generic, crises are irrelevant to "community" psychology and should be excluded from the conceptual framework.

These considerations lead in turn to the second approach, spatial extension with regard to crisis *reactions*. The locus of crisis and of disruption of equilibrium can be identified as ranging from the individual to each of the successively broad communities of which he is a member. Interest may be restricted to crises at any one level or expanded to a number of interrelated crises. If an attorney experiences a crisis reaction to the death of his spouse, for example, it is possible to confine the analysis to the disruption of his personal equilibrium and the processes directly leading to the restoration of an adaptive balance. On the other hand, for other purposes it may be necessary to look at the crisis that his temporary disequilibrium induces in his family, his clients, the court, the agency board on which he serves, or the county political group in which he is an officer . A total understanding of any crisis would theoretically have to take into account the reverberations of disruption of equilibrium at any point throughout all possible systems. Fortunately, in practice, the units of analysis can be operationally delimited. Nonetheless, as Mayo and Klein (1964) have indicated, awareness of the broad spatial implications of crisis can be crucial for certain kinds of understanding, particularly at community levels. The comments regarding temporal extension can be amplified in this light as well. That is, what has gone before and what follows may aid in the understanding of a current crisis just as much as behavior during that crisis may shed light on both the past and the future.

8. MANIPULABILITY OF VARIABLES

This dimension is fairly self-explanatory and simply asserts that models differ in the degree to which their variables can be manipulated. The usefulness of the model as a guide to practice is a function of this dimension. Crisis theory can be examined in relation to its implications for preventing the occurrence of crises and for affecting the outcome of crises once they have occurred. Event variables and vulnerability variables need to be considered separately.

Hazardous Events

The theory asserts that crises can be avoided by preventing the occurrence of a hazardous event or by mitigating the hazardous properties of inevitable events. Once a crisis occurs, its outcome is theoretically unrelated to the event which helped precipitate it.

Some events cannot be prevented, some need to occur if other goals are to be achieved, and still others depend for their prevention upon agreement that they are hazardous and that the means for prevention are appropriate. The first two classes of events will be discussed below under mitigating hazardous properties. As to the third, Signell (1969) has pointed out that pregnancy out of wedlock would usually be regarded as a hazardous event likely to result in crisis for many women. It is an event that can be prevented for many women by sex education, abstinence, or various means of artificial contraception. Yet acceptance of any or all of these means of prevention will vary widely from community to community. Variables which may theoretically be manipulable, therefore, are restricted in the extent to which the decision-making process in a community regarding crisis intervention is influenced.

Reduction of the hazardous qualities of events in order to prevent crisis can be approached both through altering the nature of events and by the provision of ameliorating supports. Again, either approach requires knowledge of the nature of the threat or hazard. Thus, the crisis hazard of hospitalizing a young child can be reduced by avoiding the mother-child separation and admitting both to the hospital. At the same time, making the hospital milieu less alien through decor, dress of ward personnel, and familiar toys and books is a crisis-intervention approach now taken for granted on most pediatric services.

For those hazardous events which are inevitable, such as the death of loved ones, every culture includes rituals and institutions designed to reduce crisis reactions and promote sanctioned grieving. Silverman (1967) has suggested, however, that recent trends of family dispersal, alienation and isolation in the cities, and changing religious values may have resulted in the reduction of available supports and an increased probability of bereavement crises, particularly in young widows.

Vulnerability

A crucial assertion of crisis theory is that personal vulnerability can be altered both to avoid the occurrence of crises and to control the outcome of crisis reactions. The literature on anticipatory guidance is devoted to the former kind of alteration, and that on crisis intervention to the latter. The premise on which anticipatory guidance rests is that appropriate preparation for specific aspects of hazardous events can promote adequate coping with those events and reduce the probability of crisis reactions. This approach is most appropriate at a population-at-risk level and does not insure against individual crisis reactions. It also depends upon knowledge of the threat or hazard. Thus, preparation for culture shock can reduce crisis reactions in Peace Corps volunteers, as Caplan (1964) has shown.

Once crisis states have occurred, intervention can lead to successful mastery by opening up avenues of resolution and providing support and guidance in the process. Jacobson and his associates (1968) have suggested that crisis intervention in many generic crises ordinarily is or can be provided by a variety of persons, while successful intervention in individual crises may require the services of a mental-health professional.

9. EVOLUTIONISM

Chapman describes his final category of analysis as

[a continuum between] quite static models, which attempt to explain through mechanisms that bring the behaving system back to original states of equilibrium, and, on the other hand, developmental models, which embody some scheme ... producing new dynamic situations with their own new equilibrium (Chapman, 1962, p. 322).

He analyzes disaster models in terms of two aspects of this continuum, both of which are relevant to the analysis of crisis theory. These have to do with whether or not the model concerns itself with developmental variables regarding individuals and regarding communities.

It is in the area of individual variables that the need for integrating concepts of developmental and accidental crises becomes apparent, although conceptual separation is useful in other respects. Theoretical propositions about crisis implicitly assume that both the likelihood of certain hazardous events occurring and the capacity of people to cope with these events are highly correlated with age or associated developmental criteria. These assumptions have not been spelled out, nor have comparative studies appeared to measure the amount of variance attributable to such factors.

For example, as people live longer, are forced to retire earlier, and subsist on reduced incomes, large numbers of elderly people can be expected to live in areas scheduled for redevelopment. Moreover, their decreasing ability to cope with change and increasing dependence on familiar surroundings make them particularly vulnerable to crises around relocation. This kind of premise can be evaluated in relation to other age groups, in relation to intact families versus isolates, and in relation to the differential preventive implications for the elderly.

If the developmental hypotheses regarding phase-specific crises which have been advanced by Erikson (1959) and others are predictive of the response of age-defined populations to certain kinds of hazardous events, then community psychologists need to explore and utilize this predictive value. Lindemann has said that "it is precisely this twilight zone between health and disease at times of developmental crises which is a major concern of the community" (Lindemann, 1965, p. 552).

It also seems possible, in time, for crisis theory to provide a perspective on those aspects of a community's development and organization which are predictive of ability to resolve community-level crises. Wilson (1962) has listed some features of community disorganization which are poor prognostically for coping with disaster. Efforts by Spiegel (1968) and others to identify community characteristics which help prevent riots have met with only limited success. The comparative study of different kinds of communities in these regards can help to link crisis theory with other ecological models.

CONCLUSIONS

The foregoing analysis has highlighted those trends which appear to have significance for the development of crisis theory and its relevance for community mental health. A different approach to the burgeoning literature and another format of analysis might yield still other features which are germane to the conceptualization of community problems. Nonetheless, the three questions raised in the section on Implication of the model clearly reflect the directions of theoretical refinement and research which have considerable generality. To review:

1. What kinds of events can be predicted to evoke crises in large numbers of persons?

2. What kinds of populations-at-risk can be identified, by reason of special vulnerability, in relation to events?

3. What kinds of interventions are specific for the favorable resolution of what kinds of crises?

Chapman's paradigm has yielded the following analysis of the present status of crisis theory as a conceptual model:

1. While crisis theory is fairly early in its development and in many ways descriptive rather than fully implicated, a number of consensual assumptions characterize the literature. These assumptions lead to hypotheses and tests which are serving to fill in the model.

2. Many studies are contributing to the understanding of both event properties and person characteristics which are important in the prediction and control of crises. Bridging concepts to explain the interaction of these sets of variables are less well developed.

3. Crisis theory concerns behavior during change or flux and focuses on those behavioral changes which occur concomitantly with environmental changes. Its operations are directed to naturally occurring life situations rather than laboratory situations. These features combine to put crisis theory toward the specific end of a Level of Abstraction continuum, since it does not purport to be a general theory of behavior.

4. There are different submodels to explain separate aspects of crisis: one set of variables relating to events, one to adaptation and coping, and another set of interaction variables. Variables borrowed from other theories and other social sciences can add to the

understanding, prediction, and control of crises.

5. The theoretical potential for comprehensiveness needs to be developed through more research on group crises and community crises to match the rich body of data on individual and family crises. This knowledge would, in turn, lead to the development of the usefulness of the crisis framework for broad-scale preventive intervention and for community planning.

6. Research on accidental crises by definition deals with a clearly truncated time unit and is thus relatively field-dependent and ahistorical. Nonetheless, some longitudinal investigations of recurrent crises could enhance our understanding of vulnerability and coping.

7. Most investigators have restricted the definition of crisis to a relatively limited social system, such as the individual and his immediate life space, or to a family and its interactions. Expansion of understanding could accrue from research which focused on interlocking crises in various community ecologies.

8. The cogency of crisis theory for community mental health and for community psychology is a function of its growth orientation and of the manipulability of its variables. Some crises can be avoided by preventing the occurrence of hazardous events or by mitigating the hazardous properties of inevitable events. Personal vulnerability can be altered both to prevent unnecessary crises and to control the outcome of crisis reactions. Tests of these kinds of manipulability are increasingly providing data to answer the three basic questions referred to above.

9. While conceptualizations of accidental crises need to be separated from those of developmental crises, each theoretical approach would be enriched through rapprochement with the implications of the other. Implicit assumptions that both the likelihood of certain hazardous events occurring and the capacity of people to cope with these events are highly correlated with age or associated developmental criteria need to be explicated and tested. Concepts of community development and organization can also aid the predictive accuracy of the crisis model and help to link crisis theory with other ecological models.

Since community psychology is a new and rapidly developing field, congenial conceptual models need to be open-ended and suggestive of new directions of investigation. This is clearly true of the present status of crisis theory. The complexity of concerns in community psychology and community mental health can be illuminated by a variety of theoretical approaches, and the task of synthesizing resultant knowledge will constitute a formidable challenge. Contributions to that knowledge, however, will continue to emerge from the highly diversified investigations which utilize concepts of crisis as a theoretical base.

REFERENCES

Barker, R. G. Explorations in ecological psychology. *Amer. Psychologist*, 1965, **20** (1), 1-14.

Bibring, Grete L., Dwyer, T. F., Huntington, Dorothy S., & Valenstein, A. F. A study of the psychological processes in pregnancy and of the earliest mother-child relationship. In Ruth S. Eissler, Anna Freud, H. Hartmann, & Marianne Kris (Eds.), *The psychoanalytic study of the child*. Vol. 16. New York: International Universities Press, 1961.

Bloom, B. C. Definitional aspects of the crisis concept. *J. consult. Psychol.*, 1963, **27** (6), 498-502.

Bowlby, J. *Maternal care and mental health*. Geneva: World Health Organization, 1952.

Caplan, G. Emotional crises. In A. Deutsch (Ed.), *The encyclopedia of mental health*. Vol. 2. New York: Franklin Watts, 1963.

Caplan, G. *Principles of preventive psychiatry*. New York: Basic Books, 1964.

Chapman, D. W. Dimensions of models in disaster behavior. In G. W. Baker & D. W. Chapman (Eds.), *Man and society in disaster*. New York: Basic Books, 1962.

Deevey, E. S. General and urban ecology. In L. J. Duhl (Ed.), *The urban condition*. New York: Basic Books, 1963.

Erikson, E. Identity and the life cycle: selected papers. *Psychol. Issues*, 1959, Vol. 1 (Whole issue).

Fried, M. Grieving for a lost home. In L. J. Duhl (Ed.), *The urban condition*. New York: Basic Books, 1963.

Hill, R. Generic features of families under stress. *Social Casewk*, 1958, **39** (2-3), 139-149.

Hirsh, J. Suicide: Part 5, The trouble shooting clinic: prototype of a comprehensive community emergency service. *Ment. Hygiene*, 1960, **44**, 496-502.

Jacobson, G. F., Wilner, D. M., Morley, W. E., Schneider, S., Strickler, M., & Sommer, G. J. The scope and practice of an early-access brief treatment psychiatric center. *Amer. J. Psychiat.*, 1965, **121** (12), 1176-1182.

Jacobson, G. F., Strickler, M., & Morley, W. E. Generic and individual approaches to crisis intervention. *Amer. J. Publ. Hlth*, 1968, **58** (2), 338-343.

Janis, I. L. *Psychological stress*. New York: Wiley, 1958.

Kalis, Betty L. The continuum of crisis. Paper presented at Symposium on Crisis Intervention and Community Mental Health, Western Psychological Association, Long Beach, California, 1966.

Kalis, Betty L., Harris, M. R., Prestwood, A. R., & Freeman, Edith H. Precipitating stress as a focus in psychotherapy. *Arch. gen. Psychiat.*, 1961, **5**, 219-226.

Kaplan, D. M., & Mason, E. A. Maternal reactions to premature birth viewed as an acute emotional disorder. *Amer. J. Orthopsychiat.*, 1960, **30** (3), 539-552.

Lazarus, R. S. *Psychological stress and the coping process.* New York: McGraw-Hill, 1966.

Lindemann, E. Symptomatology and management of acute grief. *Amer. J. Psychiat.*, 1944, **101**, 141-148.

Lindemann, E. Social system factors as determinants of resistance to change. *Amer. J. Orthopsychiat.*, 1965, **35**, 544-547.

Marks, E. S., & Fritz, C. E. Human reactions in disaster situations. Memorandum from National Opinion Research Center, 1954.

Mayo, Clara, & Klein, D. C. Group dynamics as a basic process of community psychiatry. In L. Bellak (Ed.), *Handbook of community psychiatry and community mental health.* New York: Grune & Stratton, 1964.

Mercer, Jane R. Patterns of family crisis related to reacceptance of the retardate. *Amer. J. ment. Defic.*, 1966, **71** (1), 19-32.

Miller, K. S., & Iscoe, I. The concept of crisis. *Human Organization*, 1963, **22** (3), 195-201.

Parad, H. J. (Ed.) *Crisis intervention: selected readings.* New York: Family Service Association of America, 1965.

Powell, J. W., Rayner, Jeannette, & Finesinger, J. E. Responses to disaster in American cultural groups. Paper presented at Symposium on Stress, Walter Reed Army Medical Center, Army Medical Service Graduate School, Washington, D.C., March 16-18, 1953.

Rapoport, Lydia. The state of crisis: some theoretical considerations. *Social Serv. Rev.*, 1962, **36** (2), 211-217.

Rochman, Joan. *Bibliography relating to crisis theory.* Boston: Laboratory of Community Psychiatry, Harvard Medical School, 1965.

Schulberg, H. C., & Sheldon, A. The probability of crisis and strategies for preventive intervention. *Arch. gen. Psychiat.*, 1968, **18**, 553-558.

Signell, Karen A. The crisis of unwed motherhood: a consultation approach. *Community ment. Hlth J.*, 1969, **5**, 304-313.

Silverman, Phyllis R. Services to the widowed: first steps in a program of preventive intervention. *Community ment. Hlth J.*, 1967, **3**, 37-44.

Spiegel, J. P. The functions of the scenario in collective violence. Paper presented at the Annual Meeting of the American Psychiatric Association, Boston, 1968.

Wilson R. N. Disaster and mental health. In G. W. Baker & D. W. Chapman (Eds.), *Man and society in disaster.* New York: Basic Books, 1962.

CHAPTER 6

A Role-Theory Perspective
for Community Psychology:
The Structure of Social Identity

Theodore R. Sarbin

Community psychology is a new and rapidly expanding move-ment. The psychologists who identify themselves with this new development are engaged in a wide variety of enterprises, such as reforming school curricula and administration, modifying police-community relations, identifying dysfunctional conduct in the community, reducing the incidence of violent conduct, and many more. In all such enterprises, the psychologist works as an agent of change. His efforts are in the nature of interventions, direct or indirect, designed to reorganize the conduct of selected target persons.

Being an agent of change is not a new status for psychologists. Clinical, counseling, consulting, industrial, and engineering psy-chologists, among others, have performed the role of change agents, of direct and indirect interveners, with the intention of altering the behavior of target persons. The recognition of the birth and growth of this new discipline raises this compelling question: *What differentiates the community psychologist as an agent of change from other varieties?*

The contents of this paper flow from my efforts to answer this question. *First,* I argue that the objectives of the community psy-

This chapter enlarges on some ideas first presented in 1965 at a symposium cele-brating the 20th anniversary of the Veterans Administration Mental Hygiene Clinic, Los Angeles, and later developed for an address before the Mental Health Department of Alameda County, Oakland, California, 1967. The ideas presented here served as the basis for an address to the students and faculty of Southern Illinois University, November, 1968.

chologist's interventions are unlike the objectives of other psychologists. The dissimilarity is apparent when we stand back and view the potential targets of intervention. These potential targets are different subsystems of the ecology than the targets of other psychological interveners. The community psychologist directs his efforts to a different order of events than, say, the psychotherapist, the behavior therapist, or the pastoral counselor. *Second,* I present an argument that the metaphors most congruent with the implicit thought models of the community psychologist are the metaphors of role theory. *Third,* I propose a refinement and application of role theory: the structure of social identity. I shall argue that the latter is the ultimate target of community psychologists. *Finally,* I offer some remarks about the choice of strategies of intervention —the choice being determined to a great extent by the model underlying the role metaphors.

THE INTERVENTION OBJECTIVES OF COMMUNITY PSYCHOLOGISTS

In the past, we have directed our interventions to the individual whose public conduct and/or self-evaluations were such as to lead to various forms of inefficient or dysfunctional outcomes.[1] Such outcomes are related to unsuccessful efforts by the individual to locate himself in his complicated and changing environment. For our analytical purposes, "the environment" is too coarse a construct. "The environment" may be regarded as a set of *differentiated ecologies*—that is, differentiated aspects of the world of occurrences which intrude upon man at all times and in all places. Because of space limitations, I will not discuss all these ecologies. Rather, I will focus on the assumption that man must correctly locate himself with reference to the world of occurrences in order to survive as a biosocial organism, as a valued person, as a conceptual entity, and as a member of society.[2]

The Self-Maintenance Ecology

Needless to say, to survive as a biosocial organism, man must locate himself in the self-maintenance ecology. As Darwin, among

[1] Parenthetically, tradition directs us to assign Greco-Latin labels to these persons and to call them patients. Both of these traditional labeling processes have far-reaching consequences, which I have discussed elsewhere (Sarbin, 1967, 1968b).

[2] I have developed this argument in a related paper (Sarbin, 1964a). The underlying model is described in Sarbin, Taft, & Bailey, 1960.

others, pointed out, man must be vigilant lest he become prey to ferocious beasts or to other natural perils. He must be able to answer such questions as "What is that?" and "What is next?" when he hears or sees some strange object. Since man is capable of asking questions reflexively, he may reverse the question and ask, "*What am I* in relation to the strange occurrence?" Without correct answers, his survival would be imperiled. Save for very young children, people with sensory defects, and individuals in extreme situations, most persons are able correctly to locate themselves in the self-maintenance ecology. That is to say, they are able to make discriminations between potentially hostile objects or persons and benign objects or persons. Under some conditions of ambiguity and overload, however, a person may err in his discriminations: his answers to the questions "What is it?" and "What am I?" may be mismatched to the world of occurrences. Stated in another way, he may locate himself in his ecology incorrectly, and, as a result, engage in conduct which may have disastrous consequences.

Examples of such dysfunctional conduct following upon faulty ecological discriminations would include classical phobias, overgeneralization in the use of conceptual categories, so-called hallucinations, and cognitive overinclusion. Such instances of ineffectual or dysfunctional conduct may have far-reaching consequences. The inefficiency of one individual may, for example, imperil group survival. The perpetrator of such dysfunctional conduct may then become the target of efforts designed to improve his discriminative skills. If he is considered hopeless, he may be removed from membership in the group. A segment of such persons whose discriminative skills are wanting are dispatched to mental hospitals and labeled schizophrenic. Another segment may be identified by agents of the educational system and labeled retarded or mentally deficient.

Some experimental work in progress indicates that to locate oneself in the self-maintenance ecology by answering the question "What is it?" (usually through giving answers to the reflexive "What am I?"), a person tends to use words denoting species or "thing" categories and words denoting dispositions or qualities. Examples of the latter are "I am evil," "I am strong as an ox," "I am clean." Examples of the former are "I am a sentient creature," "I am a human being," "I am a piece of clay," "I am a stone," "I am a pot," and so on. Shakespeare's Lear highlighted the problem of nonplacement in the self-maintenance ecology when he cried out, "Who is it that can tell me what I am?"

The Social Ecology

In addition to his efforts to locate himself in the self-maintenance ecology, a human being must locate himself in the social ecology—that is, the role system. The basic process of locating oneself in the social structure is an inferential one: If the person has some knowledge of the role system, then on the basis of cues available he infers the role of others and simultaneously of self. One way of communicating the essence of the process of locating the self in the social ecology is in the efforts of the person to answer the question "Who am I?" This is achieved by his answering the reflexive question "Who are you?" Establishing one's place in the social system is a relativistic, reciprocal affair: The answer to the question "Who am I?" is determined through answers to the question "Who are you?" and vice versa. *The matrix of such answers, usually in role-related terms, defines one's social identity.*

Since we live in a multiplex culture where identity is not automatically established, a person is constantly called upon to answer "Who are you?" questions. Common examples come to mind readily: when meeting strangers, when applying for employment, when seeking admission to a voluntary organization, or when taking out a marriage license, a person must establish his identity through providing his name, age, sex, marital status, occupation, memberships, education, religious affiliation, and the like.

These answers are drawn from the dimensions of the role system; they are the most convenient ways of answering the question "Who are you?" Such answers are empty, however, if they are not supported by actual or symbolic interaction with occupants of complementary statuses. For a man validly and convincingly to establish his identity as a foreman, for example, requires that he engage in appropriate supervisory behavior with reference to line workers. For a woman validly to declare her identity as a mother requires that she perform certain customary conduct with reference to sons and daughters. For a man validly to identify as a husband requires performances vis-à-vis his wife, according to the standards of his social reference groups. At any time, an individual's social identity is made up of all the social statuses that he has occupied and made good in the eyes of relevant others. A person's social identity depends upon the degree of match between his performances and the expectations held by his relevant audiences.

Regardless of whether we are interested in the observer's inferences about a person's social identity or in the subject's inferences, the point of origin is in the overt role performances and the valuations that are placed on these performances by relevant others. That is to say, both the observer and the subject may construct inferences about the subject's identity. Their conclusions may not be the same, but both shape their inferences out of the overt performances of the subject in trying to make good his role assignments.

Since role relationships are the definers of a man's social identity, planned or unplanned changes in role relationships will produce changes in the answers to the "Who are you?" questions and in the concurrent inferences about social identity. When a person fails correctly to locate himself in the social ecology, his subsequent conduct may not meet the expectations of others who have made contrary locations.

The Normative Ecology

Related to the social structure is the normative ecology—the systems of norms and values that guide cultural participation and, to a large extent, supersede specific roles. To locate himself in this ecology, it is as if a person asks, *"How well* am I meeting the standards? *How well* am I enacting a particular role? *How well* am I participating in my culture?" The answers to such questions may lead to self-evaluations of failure, disappointment, badness, loss of self-esteem or self-respect, and/or judgments by others of impropriety or inappropriateness. In the course of locating himself in the normative ecology, the individual may locate the "cause" of his proper or improper conduct within himself or external to himself. A more extended treatment of the normative ecology would lead us into a consideration of the concepts "locus of control" and "responsibility."

The Transcendental Ecology

The fourth ecology, the transcendental ecology—and the final one for this discussion—is derived from the first. While the self-maintenance ecology contains concrete objects and happenings in the physical world of occurrences, the transcendental ecology contains abstractions. The question is phrased, "What am I in relation to transcendental objects?"—God, the universe, mankind, justice, departed ancestors, and so on. Each culture has its own transcendental abstractions, and every man who participates in his culture must place himself with reference to such abstractions. Failure to find satisfactory answers to these questions may lead to chronic doubt, obsessive thought, and to other forms of conduct that interfere with individual adjustment and life.

Summary of Ecologies

If a person fails to locate himself correctly in his various ecologies, his conduct is likely to be dysfunctional, that is, inappropriate, improper, and/or ineffective. Such dysfunctional conduct may strain the tolerance limits of relevant others in his community. Traditionally, members of organized collectivities seek to neutralize the effects of dysfunctional conduct by means of two classical forms of intervention: (1) removing the deviant, and (2) altering his conduct. In general, such individuals first are referred to specialists whose aim is to assess the probability of improving conduct through therapeutic intervention before removal from the community.

To anticipate somewhat and to tie the preceding statements to subsequent remarks: Dysfunctional conduct is related to problems experienced by persons in their efforts to locate themselves in various ecologies. For any troubled person, the antecedents of dysfunctional conduct may be sought in the unanswered or incorrectly answered ecological questions. The intervention of others (shamans, psychiatrists, social workers, gurus, clergymen) is required to find proper, functional answers to ecological questions. The forms of intervention prescribed should follow from the type of ecology in which the individual mislocates himself. The targets of psychologists' (and others') interventions may be found everywhere. However, they may be sorted according to the fourfold system based on the notion of misplacement in differentiated ecologies. Furthermore, treatments and other interventions are specific to certain ecologies and not to others; for example, conduct subsequent to misplacement in the social or role ecology is the focus of interest to community psychologists, but not to behavior therapists.

ROLE THEORY AND COMMUNITY PSYCHOLOGY

The many intervention perspectives currently in fashion may be conveniently sorted into four classes. These perspectives are statements of beliefs, the origins of which are in part a function of the particular metaphors selected to denote the phenomena under scrutiny. Further, I shall assert that in the natural history of science, metaphors may become illicitly transformed to myths, and that each metaphor or myth contains implications for further theory development, for research, and for treatment (Sarbin, 1964a, 1968b).

I use the word *metaphor* in the general sense: a word borrowed from one idiom or system of discourse to denote an event appropriate to another idiom or system of discourse. For example, when Mesmer first used the term *magnetism* to denote his observations, he borrowed the term to express a similarity between events subsumed under the physical-science term, magnetism, and the events he noticed in his attempts to heal his patients. The choice of any metaphor is conditioned by concurrent scientific, political, and literary happenings available to the investigator. The person who employs the metaphor does so at first with the explicit assumption that the two events are not identical, only that there are some similarities between the observed events and the events connected with the borrowed term. For Mesmer, the explicit assumption would be of the form "It is *as if* a magnetic force were responsible for the cure of my patients." For Bleuler, "It is *as if* certain parts of the mind were split off from one another."

Whenever the observations are puzzling to the scientist (or to the man in the street, for that matter) he tries to fill the gap in his thinking by using whatever scientific or magical principles are handy.[3] When he notices similarities, he constructs an analogy and then uses the term from the analogue to describe the puzzling observations; he thus coins a metaphor. However, the metaphor may be submerged when, for various reasons, the *as if* term is dropped from discourse and resemblance is transformed to identity. In this way a myth is begun. Thus, the sentence "It is *as if* a magnetic force were operating" was illicitly changed to "It *is* a magnetic force operating," and the myth of animal magnetism was born. The sentence "It is *as if* the intellect were split off from the affect" became "The intellect *is* split off from the affect," and the

[3]This point is further amplified in Scheibe & Sarbin, 1965.

stage was set for developing the myth of schizophrenia.

Perspectives of intervention, then, are systems of metaphors and myths regarding who should be "treated" and how the treatment should be carried out. Metaphors are useful devices; they encourage us to examine old problems under a new light. Myths, on the other hand, tend to freeze conceptual and methodological approaches to problems.

With this introduction, let us look at four formulations of conduct change. Each is based on a system of metaphors, some of which have achieved mythic status: (1) behavior theory, (2) psychodynamic theory, (3) the humanist-existential viewpoint, and (4) the viewpoint of community psychology. I might add that these classes are somewhat arbitrarily formed from a larger catalogue of treatment. I grant that overlap in perspectives is the rule. My concern is the main emphases and recognizable trends.

The Perspective of Behavior Theory

The first orientation may be characterized in various ways: habit training, conditioning therapy, and behavior therapy are some of the labels. The origin of this perspective is lost in antiquity; the distinguishing feature is the recognition that environmental stimuli may direct behavior and that such stimuli may have cue properties and/or reinforcement properties. Habits may be fixed or modified by the effects of externally instigated behavior in the form of need satisfaction or tension reduction, or by the reinforcing effects of gestural and verbal behaviors of certain other persons. The underlying imagery of traditional learning theory is man-as-machine. The metaphors of the recent behavior theorists had their origin in the physiological laboratory; they regarded behavior as if it could be codified into stimuli and responses. Like the subject in the learning experiment, the behavior therapist's client or patient is treated not as a sentient, construing person, but as if he were a passive, neutral organism.

Several recent books (Krasner & Ullmann, 1965; Ullmann & Krasner, 1965; Wolpe et al., 1964) witness the now widespread use of methods based on the manipulation of objects and persons in the patient's immediate environment. The results are indeed impressive. However, one notes that behavior therapy is most successful in the changing of habits. This is not to ignore the reports that attitudes and beliefs—as expressed verbally—may be changed through the judicious scheduling of reinforcements. The behavior therapist sets out to change a specific habit or to replace one habit with another. The strict behavior therapist is unconcerned with possible changes in self-evaluations, in identity transformation, or in other abstract properties.

The early metaphors, stimulus and response, were drawn from physiological experiments and were compatible with the myth of man-as-machine. They were convergent with Darwin's notion of survival: To discriminate between threatening and benign stimuli and to make the correct response were necessary for maintaining the self. It would appear that behavior therapy would be the treatment of choice for dysfunctional conduct arising from misplacement in the self-maintenance ecology—recognizing, of course, that the self-maintenance ecology of contemporary human beings is more complex than Darwin's jungle. That is to say, the targets of behavior therapists would be the problems connected with the faulty acquisition of discriminative habits that mediate commerce with the self-maintenance ecology.

The Perspective of Psychodynamic Theory

The root metaphor of the psychodynamic perspective is *mind* or *psyche,* originally employed to denote behavior, some parts of which had covert characteristics. "Minding" was made over into a substantive by earlier authorities, reified into an invisible entity with dynamic properties, and regarded as coordinate with the body as a mechanical entity. The basic belief was founded on the metaphysical notion that there are two entities—a body and a mind—and that each can be considered independent of the other. The dualistic myth, colorfully labeled as the ghost-in-the-machine (Ryle, 1949) was founded on theological beliefs and has served as the basis for theorizing for three hundred years or more. Freud and others used this myth as the framework for theories of conduct. Many metaphors have been coined to point to similarities between known events and observation—the structure of the mind, psychic energy, Oedipus complex, hydraulic displacement, and others. The implication of this viewpoint is that disordered conduct or personal discomfort follows from imbalances or accidents to the invented structure of the mind.[4]

---

[4]The continuity of the psychodynamic perspective with Galenic medicine is apparent. The aim of Galenic practitioners was to establish harmony among the humors (Sarbin, 1968a; Sarbin & Juhasz, 1967).

But how to adjust and rearrange the mental structures? On the assumption that the talk of patients or clients contains clues about the mental mysteries, the healing art of the psychotherapist became dependent upon verbal communication. Since the mind or psyche is, by definition, immaterial, one must employ immaterial processes—and these processes were to be revealed somehow in the verbal and gestural behavior of the client. In endorsing the position that, in principle, persons could alter the structure of the mind (the causal entity in behavior) upon the completion of guided self-analysis, the psychodynamic healers implied that the individual was responsible for his own misery and suffering. If the aim of the psychodynamic therapist was to teach the client to accept responsibility for his discomfort, then the healer became, in spite of himself, a moralist (Rieff, 1961). Behind the therapist's oft-proclaimed neutrality and objectivity may be found an operative set of norms that ineluctably directs him to transmit to the client that, in the last analysis, one must take responsibility for his own hangups. When the client has difficulty, for example, in answering the ecological question "How well am I meeting my expectations of self?" his beliefs may be shaped so that his discomfort is regarded as a result of the application of his own norms to his conduct. He is faced, then, with a three-choice decision: (1) modifying or repudiating his conduct, (2) changing his norms, his value orientations, or (3) continuing to feel guilty, depressed, unhappy, uncomfortable.

The implications of this perspective for treatment are transparent. When the person has difficulty in placing himself in the normative ecology, then psychotherapy directed toward more functional placement is the treatment of choice. In order to participate in this form of treatment, the troubled person must be able to express his beliefs and understandings in sentences which, when interpreted through the prevailing mythology, give rise to such concepts as emotional health, anxiety, guilt feelings, transference, and resistance. Such treatment will continue to be useful if the metaphors are not submerged, not frozen into mythical entities, but rather regarded as ways of talking about locations in the normative ecology.

The Humanistic-Existential Perspective

Called by Maslow the "third force" in psychology, this relatively recent perspective has introduced such basic concepts as being, awareness, experience, authenticity, existential crises, and self-actualization.[5] Arguments may be presented to show that in this orientation, efforts are made to penetrate meanings that have become disguised through the use of metaphors. Just as the psychodynamic perspective had its origin in Galenic medicine, and the behavioristic perspective had its origin in laboratory physiology, so the existential perspective had its origin in humanistic philosophy and theology. The relation of man to God, of man to man, of man to nature, of being to becoming—these are the kinds of ecological issues that must be resolved. The failure satisfactorily to answer, for example, the transcendental question "What am I in relation to God?" may lead to consequences often judged deviant by relevant others. Unlike the behavior-theory and psychodynamic perspectives, treatment does not specifically require the intervention of therapists or behavior engineers. Solitude, meditation, prayer, esthetic experiences, pain and suffering may reorganize a person's relationship to ecological events of a transcendental sort. In so doing, of course, his construct of self changes correlatively with changes in construing the "eternal truths" of the transcendental ecology.

There is no paucity of claims that ours is an age of alienation, of meaninglessness, of continuing existential threat of H-bombs, of moral decay, and so on. To the extent that such claims have validity, to that extent will the existential orientation be useful. As a form of intervention, however, limitations are apparent. The kinds of clients described in Bugental's (1964) book are well-educated, abstractly intelligent middle-class persons. It is an open question whether one's relation to transcendental figures and entities is salient to miseducated, unassimilated lower-class members of racial minorities (whose existential problems stem primarily from their efforts to locate the self in the social ecology).

[5] I am aware that the historical roots of humanism and the schools of existentialism are not necessarily compatible. In the interest of brevity, however, I am using as the model for the "third force" the writings of Maslow (1962), Bugental (1965), and the recent work of Rogers and Stevens (1967).

The Perspective of Community Psychology

The fourth perspective, at least for behavioral scientists, is the most recent. As yet, it is not an organized body of knowledge, nor has it prophets or disciples. Although the labels "community psychiatry" and "community mental health" are becoming more familiar, they do not carry the meaning I intend. The extension of psychiatry to the community does not remove the medical orientation and the search for complexes and illnesses reflected by symptoms. Mental-health terms have been separated from their metaphoric origins, so that we are expected uncritically to believe that (1) there is a mind, and (2) like the body, the mind can be healthy or unhealthy. Not to get caught up in futile mentalistic metaphors, then, I use the term "community psychology" to denote an approach to intervention that differs markedly from the previously mentioned perspectives. The targets are organizations of persons whose conduct is dysfunctional as a result of ecological misplacement or nonplacement. To rephrase my earlier statement, the social ecology may profitably be conceptualized as a system of role relationships. In this context, the metaphors of role theory are continuous with the rationale of community psychology.[6]

Role Concepts

The term *role* is borrowed directly from the theater. Auxiliary metaphors include role-taking skill, the complementarity of conduct, congruence of self and role, convincingness of enactment, and others. Role is a metaphor intended to denote that conduct adheres to certain "parts" or positions rather than to the players who read or recite their parts. In the etymology of the word *role*, there is a historical continuity not usually found in psychological or psychiatric vocabularies. The root of the term referred to the roller about which a parchment was rolled and from which the actor read his part. The antecedent to the writing and later reciting and acting of such parts was, and is, the conduct of real-life human beings struggling to make their way in imperfectly organized societies. Thus, there exists a metaphorical continuity from social life to dramatic portrayals on stage, and from the dramatic idiom to psychological theory concerned with social beings enacting real-life dramas.

[6]For a recent paper on the place of role theory in current psychology, see my chapter in Worchel and Byrne (1964b) and Sarbin and Allen (1968).

This perspective addresses itself to the role enactments of persons in social settings. To interpret conduct as role enactment immediately places constraints on methods of observation and analysis. The focus of attention is on *overt* social conduct. Questions of this sort arise: What are the positions or statuses of the others toward whom the actor is performing? What are the obvious and subtle contributions of others to the enactment—are they providing rewards and punishments, are they informing, are they contradictory?

Unlike other interventions, role enactment bridges the gap between the individual and his society, between personal history and social organization. The exclusive focus on the individual per se is out of place here. Rather, the focus is on the individual as a member of a collectivity, acting and interacting with others. In order to perform effectively and appropriately, the actor must accurately place himself in the role ecology, that is, he must be able to answer continually emerging questions of the "Who am I?" sort. Failure to do so through lack of clarity in role expectations, through contradictory role demands, and so on may lead to dysfunctional conduct. It follows that diagnostic and treatment efforts must be directed not to the arbitrarily isolated "patient," but rather to the relevant role set—to the relevant others in the social ecology.

A MODEL OF SOCIAL IDENTITY

To provide a theoretical background for community psychology, I present a sketch of a three-dimensional model of conduct—an outgrowth of role theory. The basic construct is social identity, a cognitive outcome that follows from an actor's conduct *and* the evaluations declared by relevant others on such conduct.

The model follows from the basic postulate that human beings constantly strive to locate themselves in their various ecologies. In order to make efficient choices from among behavior alternatives, a person must locate himself with regard to the world of occurrences. As I said before, the world may be differentiated into a number of ecologies, among them the social ecology or role system. Constantly faced with the necessity of locating himself, a person's misplacement of self in the role system may lead to embarrassing, perilous, or even fatal consequences.

Locating oneself in the role system follows from an inferential process: On the basis of clues available and of his knowledge of the role system, the individual infers the roles of others and concurrently of self. The process of locating self and others is concisely expressed as the efforts of a person to find answers to the question "Who am I?"

Answers to such questions are drawn from the categories of the role system. It is important to note that all role categories imply relationships: there can be no role of teacher without the complementary role of student; no role of mother without the role of child; and so on. Further, such relationships are imbedded in the social systems in which the person operates.

Since role relationships are the definers of one's social identity, planned or unplanned changes in role relationships will alter the answers to the "Who are you?" questions and the simultaneous inferences about social identity. Changes in social identity are the rule, occurring with changes in the roles of complementary others; for example, one's location in social space is different when he interacts with an adult or with a child, with a policeman or with a physician, with a friend or with a stranger. To understand the conduct of a participant in our culture, it is necessary to construct a set of dimensions that makes it possible to determine the relative contribution of *particular roles* to one's social identity. Further, these dimensions should facilitate recognition of the effects of intentional or unintentional shifting of one's placement in the role system. For this purpose, I make use of a three-dimensional model that provides the means for assessing the total value of a person's social identity at any point in time (Sarbin, Scheibe, & Kroger, 1965; Sarbin, 1967). The three dimensions are (1) the status dimension, (2) the value dimension, and (3) the involvement dimension. Hopefully, the suitability of this model as a candidate to displace the entrenched mental-illness model will become apparent during the following exposition.

The Status Dimension

In discussing the first dimension, we shall use the term *status* in the sociological sense of being equivalent to "position in a social structure." The relationship between role and status is governed by the conventional definitions: a status or position is an abstraction defined by the expectations held by members of the relevant society; role is a set of behaviors enacted by an individual in connection with his efforts to make good his occupancy of a particular status or position. Another way of differentiating these related concepts is to regard position or status as a cognitive notion, a set of expectations that is carried around in one's head; and to regard role as a unit of conduct, characterized by overt actions. Individual differences in both the expectations and the role performances are to be expected.

Our point of departure is Linton's classification of statuses (and their corresponding roles) as ascribed or achieved. For conceptual analysis, Linton (1936) separated those statuses that are defined by biosocial characteristics (such as age, sex, and kinship), which he called *ascribed,* from those statuses characterized by attainment or option, which he called *achieved.* Common examples of ascribed statuses are mother, son, widow, orphan, adult, child, uncle, male, and female; of achieved statuses, village chief, rock-and-roll singer, and candidate for political office. This two-valued dimension is too limiting, primarily because of instances that show the contribution of both ascriptive and achievement factors. Further analysis suggests that rather than being two-valued, the dimension is a continuum. The underlying conception is the degree of choice prior to entry into any particular status. At one end point of the dimension is the status of cultural man, with sex roles, age roles, and kinship roles being in the same region. The opposite end of the dimension is defined by statuses with high degrees of choice, such as treasurer of the local P.T.A., drum major of the school marching band. Several pathways lead to the occupancy of positions heavily weighted with choice, among them, election, nomination, training, revelation, and achievement.

At the ascribed end, statuses may be further defined as granted, or culturally given, and less differentiated. The performance of these statuses generally applies to large numbers of participants in a culture. Thus, every adult member of a culture, in principle, is granted the status of cultural participant or *person;* that is, he is expected to perform, within his biological limitations, according to certain propriety norms that take priority over specific expectations attached to any achieved status. The occupant of this granted status of person is also guaranteed certain minimal rights.

At the achieved end of the continuum, statuses may be additionally defined as optional and highly differentiated, the requirements for occupying such statuses applying to a very small number of potential candidates. Examples would be a Nobel Prize winner, a Davis Cup winner, and the Secretary General of the United Nations. The dimension is highly correlated with legitimate power and/or social esteem. In addition to the bare minima of rights granted an individual by virtue of his holding the ascribed status of person, he acquires grants of legitimate power and esteem according to the location of the positions toward the achievement or choice end of the dimension. At this point, then, we can assert that the social identity we assign an individual will in general depend upon his performance of several roles located at different points on the dimension, some carrying explicit grants of power and/or esteem, others little or none.

The Value Dimension

The model takes on more meaning when we consider the second component: the value dimension. At the same time that role enactments provide the basis for an observer to locate an individual's identity on the status dimension, they provide the basis for placement on the value dimension. The value continuum is constructed orthogonally to the status continuum, with a neutral point and with positive and negative end points. The range of potential valuations, in this model, is not the same for the enactment or nonenactment of roles at different points on the status dimension.

Let us consider first the range of potential valuation to be applied to the occupancy of statuses at the achievement end: The valuations declared on nonperformance or poor performance tend to be near the neutral point. In general, negative valuations are not applied to people who fail in their attempts at validating statuses heavily weighted with choice, such as, for example, occupational and recreational statuses. Being fired from a job, dropped from a team, or dismissed from college does not enrage or perturb a community. The responses to such outcomes of nonperformance are formalized as failure, underachievement, poor judgment, or misfortune; and noted with verbal expressions of sadness, disappointment, sympathy, regret. On the other hand, the *proper* performance of role behaviors at the choice end earns tokens of high positive value, such as Nobel prizes, public recognition, monetary rewards, and other indicators of esteem. The range of valuation for role enactments that validate achieved statuses is represented in the model as neutral to positive.

Let us consider next the range of potential valuation to be declared on role enactments designed to validate statuses that are primarily ascribed or granted. Little or no positive value is assigned to individuals for the enactment of granted roles. An individual is not praised for participation in a culture as a male, an adult, a father, a person. One is expected to enact such roles without positive public valuations. The *nonperformance* of such roles, however, calls out strong negative valuations. Consider the valuations made when a male fails to perform according to the expectations for masculine sexuality; consider the sanctions imposed when a mother fails to be interested in the care and welfare of her children; consider the value judgments rendered upon people who fail to act according to entrenched age standards; consider the value assigned to a man who publicly insults his father. The status of *person*—the very end point of the first dimension—carries with it expectations that the status occupant will engage in role behavior to meet minimal cultural expectations. Conceptualized as propriety norms, these expectations are concerned with reciprocal social interaction (communication), modesty, property, and ingroup aggression. When these role requirements are perceived as being violated, the individual holding the minimal granted position is negatively valued and marked with a pejorative label. Many forms of the label may be identified; they all denote the social identity of a *nonperson.* That is to say, if the pejorative label is applied, then the society goes to work to treat the individual as if he were not a person. The concept most widely used to represent nonperson is brute, sometimes rendered as beast, animal, or low-grade human (Sarbin, 1967; Platt & Diamond, 1965). The reason such labels are not a part of our scientific and professional lexicon is that we have coined special euphemisms which conceal only a small part of the strong negative valuational component—for example, slum dwellers, low-class, disadvantaged, foreigners, rabble, underprivileged, charity cases, paupers, mentally ill, welfare recipients, problem families, patients, wards. These labels carry much of the meaning of nonperson; the labeled individual is likely to be handled as if he were without grade on the first dimension and with negative value on the second. The pejorative labels provide a means of answering simultaneously the "Who am I?" question and the "Who are you?" question by establishing for the "you" a degraded social identity.

The valuation dimension is further developed elsewhere (Sarbin et al., 1965). Positive valuations appear to fit the semantic space occupied by the conventional expression esteem. Thus, performance of choice roles may be located on a scale from little esteem to high esteem. Nonperformance of choice roles receives a neutral valuation, that is, zero degree of esteem. Negative valuations fit the semantic space occupied by "disrespect" or "no respect." The public nonperformance of granted roles results in taking away from an individual the respect that inheres in the associated status. Motherhood is respected until the occupant of the position of mother fails to meet expectations of the group insofar as providing care for her children. The performance of granted roles, however, earns no special tokens of respect (or of esteem). One is expected to perform granted roles without incentive motivations; disrespect and associated negative sanctions follow nonperformance.

The Involvement Dimension

The third component, also a continuum, considers the involvement or engrossment or degree of participation of self in the role enactment. Any role may be enacted with various degrees of involvement, and may be recognized in at least two ways: (1) the *amount of time* a person spends in occupying a status calling for certain role enactments relative to other statuses, and (2) the *degree of organismic energy* expended in the performance. An individual whose identity includes a status at the achievement end of the continuum may be highly involved in the associated role enactment part of the time, and not involved at other times. In short, there is variation in time and energy expended in enacting chosen roles. A baseball star may be highly involved in his role when on the diamond, when in training, when reviewing batting averages. He may be relatively uninvolved in the baseball-player role when attending a funeral, when writing letters, or when visiting friends. At the ascribed or granted end, involvement is typically high; that is, there is little variation in that the actor is required to be "in role" most of the time. To be cast in the role of adult female, for example, means being "on" almost continuously. To be cast in the role of old man similarly demands high involvement. To be cast solely in the extreme granted role of person, or its negatively valued counterpart, nonperson, similarly means being in role (on stage) all the time. Examples of roles which are highly involving and with limited choice components are prisoners in maximum-security institutions, committed inmates of state mental hospitals, and unemployed workers in urban ghettos.

In the world of work, involvement in the occupational role varies with the speed and complexity of the job demands. The degree of involvement is reduced when the work flow stops—during coffee breaks, during lunch periods. In the relatively totalistic setting of the prison, the mental hospital, or the culture of poverty, for the captive, the patient, or the pauper respectively, opportunities for variation in involvement are restricted. In these settings, involvement in roles heavily weighted with ascriptive features is typically high—not by choice, but by the demands of the total situation. In short, the social identity of a member of these classes of persons does not include achieved roles, the enactment of which may be cyclical. Legitimate opportunities for obtaining role distance, in Goffman's (1961) terms, are absent when one's identity is composed exclusively of granted roles.

Parenthetically, it is interesting to speculate about the kinds of motivational theories suggested to account for the nonperformance of granted roles and for the nonperformance of chosen roles. The latter case is seldom taken as a starting point for elaborating a causal theory. When an athletic champion loses his title, a corporation executive is demoted, or a politician fails to win an election, explanations are drawn from rule-following models. Failure is attributed to lack of practice, aging, superior competition, economic considerations, and the like. The nonperformance of granted roles, however, calls out explanations of a causal kind, such as heredity, somatotypes, unconscious conflicts, toxins, psychic forces, psychosexual complexes, and so on.

Summary of Social-Identity Dimensions

An individual's social identity can be assessed by noting the statuses he occupies, the valuations placed on his performance or nonperformance of these statuses, and the degree of involvement in the roles enacted. Every status may be located on a dimension based on degree of choice prior to entry into that status. One pole of the dimension is ascribed or granted; the other, achieved or chosen. Neutral valuations are declared on highly involving role performances, if appropriate, to validate granted statuses; negative valuations, if inappropriate. No valuations are legitimately possible if involvement is nil.

THE UPGRADING AND DEGRADING
OF SOCIAL IDENTITY

This sketch of a theoretical model provides the conceptual tools for understanding both positive and negative forms of identity transformation. Mention may be made of the implications of *positive* identity transformations. Under the label of upgrading, two general classes of social process may be identified. The first, *promotion*, provides individuals with increased numbers of statuses that are characterized by choice or achievement. The second, *commendation*, provides opportunities for applying positive values to the enactment of granted roles. The process of upgrading is the reverse of degrading, the negative transformation of social identity—about which more needs to be said.

People with degraded social identities are the potential, if not the actual, candidates for the helping services, welfare actions, psychological and social interventions. From the preceding remarks, it would follow that to degrade an individual's social identity, one need only remove from him the opportunity to enact roles that have elements of choice. The more one's identity is made up of granted roles, the fewer opportunities he has of engaging in role behavior that may be positively valued. The best he can hope for is to be neutrally valued (not disrespected) through the proper, appropriate, and convincing enactment of his granted roles, all of which are highly involving. It is obvious that such a state of affairs could be achieved, it at all, only at the expense of high degrees of strain. And the maximum possible reward would be a neutrally valued social identity. It is a legitimate question whether the payoffs are commensurate with the high degree of strain imposed on the individual. It is no wonder that indices of social pathology are highest among populations that exhibit these characteristics. If, let us say, we take away a man's job and other vehicles for achieving a positively valued identity, he has few chances of displaying conduct that may be esteemed by self or others. The difference is one of degree between this example and the more commonly used examples of degraded identities: inmates in a maximum-security prison, patients in locked wards of mental hospitals, and prisoners of war in thought-control camps. The totalistic social organization of these examples leads to degradation *in extremis*, to the identity of nonperson.

The differences in degree between these totalistic settings and the settings that provide potential candidates for helping services is reflected in the fact that the relevant societies are not completely totalistic. During their early socialization experiences, these potential candidates acquire beliefs that they may someday perform roles-by-choice and thus attain a valued social identity. First in the bosom of the family, then in the early years of school, then through the mass media, the child is led to believe that he has a chance of occupying statuses that have achieved as well as granted components. Such a system of beliefs might be elided into the following shorthand premise: "In addition to being a person, male, son, I am a worthy and valued member of society." Relevant and significant others in the social ecology, however, withhold confirming positive valuations because the individual does not in fact occupy achieved statuses. A contrary premise is thus formed: "I am not a worthy and valued member of society." Such paired contrary premises are the conditions of cognitive strain—a state of affairs for which the common word *problem* is a more felicitous expression than *sickness.*

How does one go about reducing cognitive strain, solving the problem created by the contrary premises? Restrictions are imposed on the form and content of problem solving parallel to the restrictions in the range of values assignable to occupants of granted statuses. The social networks of individuals valued for their performances of roles-by-choice provide large numbers of avenues for reducing strain and reconciling contrary premises. The social networks of degraded individuals are limited—usually to similarly degraded human beings.

In addition, the social conditions that promote degradation also retard the development of differentiated concepts and modulated action. For example, restricted linguistic structures, external locus of control, and undifferentiated time perspective are to be found in the quasi-totalistic cultures of poverty (Sarbin, 1967). For this reason, the employment of universal adaptive techniques to reduce strain, to find solutions to problems, tends to be more extreme among degraded people. Their use of instrumental acts to change their relationship with the distal ecologies, for example, tends to be unmodulated by verbal controls. Thus, they are diagnosed as agitators, extremists, or unrealistic revolutionaries. Their use of the releasing powers of unregulated motor activity (as in spontaneous dancing) is characteristically without strong social or verbal controls. Such conduct conventionally receives a diagnosis of "acting out." Their use of the tranquilizing features of sleep, sex, and drugs also tends toward the extreme, and they are labeled as escapists. Their use of superordinate belief systems to reconcile contrary premises tends to be messianic, fundamentalistic, and highly personalized. They are labeled superstitious or delusional or schizophrenic.

IMPLICATIONS OF THE MODEL

The implications of this model—designed to displace the entrenched medical model—are transparent. In the first place, our case-finding techniques would be guided by a theory of social identity and the socially dysfunctional outcomes of degradation. That is to say, we would try to locate those individuals and groups whose efforts to establish acceptable social identities have been unsuccessful. These persons would show the characteristics of degraded identities, as indicated before.

Past efforts at case finding have been built on implicit psychiatric criteria (Srole et al., 1962; Leighton et al., 1963). Nontreated cases have been discovered in the sampled communities who appear to be as "sick" as persons in treatment or in mental hospitals. *Sickness* is defined by inferences based on the notion of self-reported correlates of an ambiguous mental state called "anxiety." The scientific status of "anxiety" as the basis for "sickness" is questionable (Sarbin, 1964a, 1968a). Many of these "sick" respondents who show signs of "anxiety" were functioning effectively.

Rather than continue the use of such implicit psychiatric criteria, I have explored the possibilities of a case-finding procedure based on the notion of degraded social identities. A conduct-impairment scale was developed on the explicit assumption that individuals can describe themselves in ways that reflect the valuations declared by others. Such self-description is implemented through the use of a scale made up of 58 items. The current study compares the responses of patients in treatment with responses of a matched nontreated sample: 40 items of this Conduct Impairment Scale indicate whether the respondent sees himself as a degraded, devalued individual; 18 items indicate self-characterizations that presumably reflect prolonged *effects* of occupying nonvalued statuses. Illustrative of the first category are the following items:

Most people who know me respect me as a person. *False*
There are times when I question who I really am. *True*
I always have plenty of interesting things to do. *False*

Illustrative of the second category are these items:

I very frequently feel that people are critical of my appearance and behavior. *True*
It's a good thing that a person can get lost in his thoughts and free himself from hopelessness. *True*
The most important people in my life are the ones who least understand me. *True*

The scale correctly classified 75 per cent of the sample.

In addition to providing a fresh approach to case finding, the implications of the social-identity model for intervention are transparent. Community psychologists must learn to recognize the process of degradation as it occurs and to set up procedures for giving the potentially disturbed and disturbing individuals opportunities for being positively valued. Particularly useful is the concept of role set (Merton, 1957; Kahn et al., 1964). Social and psychological intervention is directed toward social subsystems, toward *all* persons enacting interrelated roles, the value-declarers as well as the degraded persons. The community psychologist, then, must be sensitive to the fact that the "social systems" approach is more likely to achieve his goals than "psyche systems."

SUMMARY

In writing a role-theoretical perspective for community psychology, my first task was to differentiate the actions and potential actions of community psychologists from the actions of other change agents. This task led to a recognition of the fact that there are multiple targets for change agents, these targets being conceptualized as the conduct of persons in differentiated ecologies. For the purposes of this exposition, four ecologies were identified: the self-maintenance ecology, the social ecology, the normative ecology, and the transcendental ecology. In the body of the paper, I offered arguments to suggest that the targets of behavior therapists are the discriminative habits of persons who mislocate themselves in the self-maintenance ecology; the targets of psychodynamically oriented therapists are the cognitive constructions of persons who mislocate themselves in the normative ecology; the targets of humanist-existential therapists are the abstractions of persons who mislocate themselves in relation to the transcendental ecology; and the targets of the community psychologist are the social identities of persons who mislocate themselves in the social (or role) ecology.

The second task was to show that the metaphors of role theory, including the notion of social identity, were continuous with the aims and objectives of the newly developing field of community psychology. Toward this end, I called upon a three-dimensional model, first developed by Sarbin, Scheibe, and Kroger (1965), to offer a set of dimensions for understanding the concept of social identity. The concept is the resultant of the placement of an individual into a three-dimensional model, the dimensions of which are (1) status, (2) valuation, and (3) involvement.

The model provides a basis for clearly recognizing that social identities may be degraded. Degradation of social identity provides the basis for categorizing individuals as nonpersons—a state of affairs that facilitates nonplacement or misplacement in social systems. The efforts of community psychologists, then, are directed toward modifying "systems of relationships," the aim of which is more effective placement of target persons in the social system.

Finally, I pointed to some practical implications of the theory for case finding and for conduct reorganization. Case finding is carried out, not by relying on medical or psychiatric models, but rather on discovering those individuals whose identities have been degraded. For conduct reorganization, the problem is to identify the features of the social system that produce degraded identities and to modify such features. The theme of the role theory of conduct reorganization is expressed in the words of John Donne: "No man is an island. ..."

REFERENCES

Bugental, J. F. T. *The search for authenticity: an existential analytic approach to psychotherapy.* New York: Holt, Rinehart & Winston, 1965.

Goffman, E. *Asylums.* Chicago: Aldine, 1961.

Kahn, R., Wolfe, D. M., Quinn, R. P., Snoek, J. D., & Rosenthal, R. A. *Organizational stress: studies in role conflict and ambiguity.* New York: Wiley, 1964.

Krasner, L., & Ullmann, L. P. *Research in behavior modification: new developments and implications.* New York: Holt, Rinehart & Winston, 1965.

Leighton, Dorothea C., Harding, J. S., Macklin, D. B., Macmillan, A. M., & Leighton, A. H. *The character of danger: psychiatric symptoms in selected communities.* Vol. 3, *The Stirling County study of psychiatric disorder and sociocultural environment.* New York: Basic Books, 1963.

Linton, R. *The study of man.* New York: D. Appleton-Century, 1936.

Maslow, A. *Toward a psychology of being.* Princeton, N.J.: Van Nostrand, 1962.

Merton, R. *Social theory and social structure.* (2nd ed.) Glencoe, Ill.: Free Press, 1957.

Platt, A. M., & Diamond, B. L. The origins and development of the wild beast concept of mental illness and its relation to theories of criminal responsibility. *J. Hist. behav. Sci.,* 1965, 1, 355-367.

Rieff, P. *Freud: the mind of the moralist.* New York: Doubleday, 1961.

Rogers, C., & Stevens, B. *Person to person: the problem of being human.* Walnut Creek, Calif.: Real People Press, 1967.

Ryle, G. *The concept of mind.* New York: Barnes & Noble, 1949.

Sarbin, T. R. Anxiety: reification of a metaphor. *Arch. gen. Psychiat.,* 1964, 10, 630-638. (a)

Sarbin, T. R. Role-theoretical interpretation of psychological change. In P. Worchel & D. Byrne (Eds.), *Personality change.* New York: Wiley, 1964. (b)

Sarbin, T. R. The dangerous individual: an outcome of social identity transformations. *Brit. J. Criminol.,* 1967, 7, 285-295.

Sarbin, T. R. Notes on the transformation of social identity. In L. Roberts, N. Greenfield, & M. Miller (Eds.), *Comprehensive mental health: the challenge of evaluation.* Madison: Univer. of Wisconsin Press, 1968. (a)

Sarbin, T. R. Ontology recapitulates philology: the mythic nature of anxiety. *Amer. Psychologist,* 1968, 23, 411-418. (b)

Sarbin, T. R. The culture of poverty, social identity and cognitive outcomes. In V. L. Allen (Ed.), *Psychological factors in poverty.* Chicago: Markham, 1969.

Sarbin, T. R., & Allen, V. L. Role theory. In G. Lindzey & E. Aronson (Eds.), *Handbook of social psychology.* Reading, Mass.: Addison-Wesley, 1968.

Sarbin, T. R., & Juhasz, J. The historical background of the concept of hallucination. *J. Hist. behav. Sci.,* 1967, 3, 339-358.

Sarbin, T. R., Scheibe, K. E., & Kroger, R. O. The transvaluation of social identity. Unpublished manuscript, 1965.

Sarbin, T. R., Taft, R., & Bailey, D. E. *Clinical inference and cognitive theory.* New York: Holt, Rinehart & Winston, 1960.

Scheibe, K. E., & Sarbin, T. R. Toward a theoretical conceptualization of superstition. *Brit. J. Phil. Sci.,* 1965, 62, 143-158.

Srole, L., Langner, T. S., Michael, S. T., Opler, M. K., & Rennie, T. A. C. *Mental health in the metropolis: the midtown Manhattan study.* New York: McGraw-Hill, 1962.

Ullmann, L. P., & Krasner, L. (Eds.) *Case studies in behavior modification.* New York: Holt, Rinehart & Winston, 1965.

Wolpe, J., Salter, A., & Reyna, L. J. (Eds.) *The conditioning therapies: the challenge in psychotherapy.* New York: Holt, Rinehart & Winston, 1964.

CHAPTER 7

Self-Valuation, Social Valuation, and Self-Identity: A Framework for Research in Social and Community Psychology

Daniel Adelson

A core problem for community psychology and community mental health is the fit between the *individual*—his capacities, expectations, aspirations, attitudes, beliefs, values—and the *community*—with its standards, norms, regulations, laws, customs, institutions, values. Central to this fit is the individual's sense of ego-identity. As Erikson has defined it:

Ego-identity is the inner capital accrued from all the experiences of each successive stage, when successful identifications led to a successful alignment of the individual's basic drives with his *endowment* and his opportunities ... The sense of ego-identity, then, is the accrued confidence that one's ability to maintain inner sameness and continuity (one's ego in the psychological sense) is matched by the sameness and continuity of one's meaning for others (Jahoda, 1958, p. 29).

A major aspect of this problem is the relation of social valuation to self-valuation and self-identity. Many of an individual's characteristics (for example, his religion, race, color, education, occupation), which form a part of his self-concept, are differentially valued by the larger majority culture, and the questions present themselves:

1. What is the relation between the cultural valuation of a significant aspect of the self and the individual's valuation of this aspect of the self?
2. What is the relation between the cultural valuation of a sig-

Revision of a paper presented at the First International Congress of Social Psychiatry, London, 1964.

nificant aspect of the self and the individual's identification with this aspect?

3. What is the relation between individual devaluation of (dislike for) a significant aspect of the self and the level of self-acceptance?

4. What is the relation between individual valuation of a significant aspect of the self and individual identification with this aspect?

A STUDY OF FIRST NAMES

A summary of an experimental exploration of these relations through a study of first names will provide an illustration of one approach to these questions (Adelson, 1964a). As previous studies (Bugental & Zelen, 1950; Duss, 1946; Hildreth, 1936; Jahoda, 1954) have shown, the first name forms a central anchorage point of the self-concept for most individuals. A series of hypotheses was developed on the basis of previous investigations of the first name, on the basis of a consideration of the nature of the self and its development (Mead, 1934; James, 1948; Murphy, 1947; Clark & Clark, 1947), and on the basis of several pilot studies. Three instruments were used to explore these hypotheses: (1) a questionnaire which included questions on attitudes toward and identification with one's own first name, among others; (2) a groupwide rating scale of first names; and (3) the self-acceptance scale developed by Berger (1952). These instruments, which were intended to measure variables at the three different levels—(1) individual attitudes and identification, (2) cultural attitudes on the dimension of liking, and (3) individual self-acceptance—were administered to 207 high-school students and 181 college students. The findings for both groups showed that:

1. Most individuals tend to like their own first names.

2. Those whose first names are liked by the group culture like their names more frequently than those whose first names are disliked by the group.

3. Individuals who dislike their own first names tend to be less self-accepting than individuals who like, or are indifferent to, their own first names.

4. Individuals who like their own first names tend to identify with the name; that is, they answer "Yes" to the question, "Do you

feel your first name is you?" more frequently than do individuals who dislike their first names.

5. Groupwide liking for the first name, however, is not related to individual identification with own name.

An analysis of the high as compared with the relatively low in self-acceptance among the 46 subjects who disliked their first names reveals that a crucial factor separating those who dislike their first names and are self-accepting from those who dislike their first names and are relatively self-rejecting is identification with own first name. In practically every instance in which there is identification *either by self or by others* with a disliked first name, there is an associated self-rejection.

On the other hand, the self-accepting individual who is identified with his own name rejects the negative "social valuation" of the larger culture, and does not express dislike for his own name in line with cultural dislike or devaluation. Thus the individual's attitudes toward his own name reflect his attitudes toward himself,[1] and depending on other factors, may or may not be in line with the cultural valuation.

AUTONOMY AND HOMONOMY

It is suggested that the positive self-valuations of the self-accepting individual depend on his sense of belonging to a smaller family, peer, or other kind of group which values his particular qualities and provides an anchor of strength in the face of majority devaluations. A sense of basic positive self-valuation is developed and nourished by the smaller group to which the individual belongs. This interpretation is supported by the views of such varied theorists as Harry Stack Sullivan, Samuel Slavson, and Andras Angyal.

Sullivan has stressed that the individual's self grows out of and is based on his interrelations with others; "the self-dynamism is built up out of this experience of approbation and disapproval, of reward and punishment" (Mullahy, 1955, p. 295).

Slavson (1943) has listed four cardinal needs, two of which are (1) the need for the unconditional love of an authority figure (which I translate as sense of belongingness in the parental family) and (2) the need for interaction with and acceptance by a peer

[1] It is also true that the name may serve as a way of selectively viewing others (Schoenfeld, 1942) or of selectively viewing self and thus influence concepts of self and of others (Adelson, 1953).

group. Slavson also lists (3) the need for a sense of self-worth and (4) the need for an interest. Slavson's views of cardinal needs may be seen as related to Angyal's postulation that there are two basic trends in man: the striving for autonomy and the striving for homonomy. Angyal has stated that "without autonomy, without self-government, the life process probably could not be understood" (Angyal, 1941, p. 34), and, further, that

At each stage of the biological process the tendency is toward a situation which is characterized by a greater degree of autonomy than the preceding situation (Angyal, 1941, p. 41).

With respect to the trend toward homonomy, Angyal notes that it "is a trend to be in harmony with superindividual units, the social group, nature, God, ethical world order" (Angyal, 1941, p. 172). These two strivings may be considered highly interrelated, and are useful concepts for interpreting such varied experiences as reactions of concentration-camp victims to extreme conditions (Adelson, 1962), or the social factors influencing placement of the chronic schizophrenic patient (Adelson, 1964b).

Various studies may be interpreted as demonstrating the interrelatedness of these two strivings. Levy's (1943) classic work on maternal overprotection may be interpreted as showing that it is possible to be more autonomous where there is a sense of belongingness which is neither rejection nor overprotection (White, 1948).

The movement of members toward more autonomous functioning in relation to the designated trainer (autonomy) and subsequently toward greater interaction with and acceptance of each other (homonomy) also seems to characterize the human-relations training group (Bennis & Shepard, 1961).

Individuals finding no belongingness (homonomy) in one group are faced with the problem of finding new groups which permit expression of their views (autonomy), as Leighton (1945) has pointed out in his study of Japanese relocation centers. The experiments described by Asch (1960) and Crutchfield (1955) may be interpreted as demonstrating this need for homonomy: when one member of a previously totally opposed group provided the correct judgment, the result was autonomy or independence of view by the formerly conforming subjects.

Being caught up in two opposed groups, on the other hand, may have disastrous consequences. One example is the secretary to the "closed ranks" investigators (Cumming & Cumming, 1957). Caught between the community of which she was a member and the research group of which she was the secretary, this woman experienced an anxiety attack. Another example is the "psychotic" breaks among the women who returned to the maternal dwelling described by Sampson and his associates (1964).

It should not be overlooked that such individual factors as physical size and appearance, education, intelligence, skill, wealth may make it easier for an individual to gain acceptance and belongingness in a group and in the community. The lack of primary family and friendship groups (homonomy) and the lack of education and skills (the possibility of autonomy and of fulfilling a function in society) are related to chronicity in schizophrenic patients (Adelson, 1964b).

APPLICATIONS OF THEORY

The theory presented here, which is based on an investigation of names, finds further support in such diverse areas of behavior as majority-minority relations, juvenile delinquency, and some manifestations of psychiatric disorder, as independently reported by different investigators.

Majority-Minority Relations

Lewin has pointed out how important for self-acceptance saying a positive "Yes" to a core aspect of self-identification may sometimes be for the minority member:

Whatever one's opinion about Zionism as a political program may be, no one who has observed closely the German Jews during the fateful first weeks after Hitler's rise to power will deny that thousands of German Jews were saved from suicide only by the famous article of the *Judische Rundschau*, with its headlines, "Jasagen zum Judentum" ("Saying Yes to Being a Jew"). The ideas expressed there were the rallying point and the source of strength for Zionist and non-Zionist alike (Lewin, 1948, p. 198).

Saying "Yes" to being a Jew in this context meant saying "No" to the wider cultural devaluation of Jews under Nazism.

The current movement toward Black Power may also be interpreted as saying a positive "Yes" to and valuing a core aspect of self-identification.

Delinquency

The same theory may be applied in an interpretation of certain types of delinquency. Cohen's theoretical approach to delinquency has been described as follows:

4. An important condition for an individual's adjustment is that he be thought well of by others who are important to him, and by himself.

5. For many working-class children, this condition is hard to fulfill. In school, in recreation centers, in all the activities of the larger community, they are judged in terms of middle-class standards, which many working-class children, for a variety of reasons, are not well-equipped to meet.

6. The delinquent subculture deals with this problem by providing criteria of status which these children can meet.

7. Since most working-class children have been exposed to, and have partially internalized middle-class standards, there is a conflict between these standards and those of the delinquent gang.

8. In order to eliminate this conflict, the delinquent subculture explicitly rejects (that is, it does not simply ignore) middle-class standards, particularly as they refer to the symbols and actuality of achieved status; the criteria for status within the delinquent gang are the opposite of those held by "respectable" society (Cohen, 1959, pp. 488-489).

Thus, the delinquent gang provides an anchorage point of strength for certain children in the conflict they face between their characteristics as they are and the negative valuation placed on these characteristics by society at large.

Neurosis

The inner conflict between the self as it is and the self as society would seem to want it to be may result in neurosis. Jung introduced the concept of the *persona* to describe such conflict.

The word "persona" is really a very suitable expression for it, since persona originally meant the mask worn by an actor to signify his role. ... It is a *compromise between the individual and society* as to the kind of semblance to adopt, what a man should "appear to be." He takes a name, earns a title, represents an office, and belongs to this or that. ... Society expects, and indeed must expect, that every individual should play the role assigned to him as completely as possible. Accordingly, a man who is also a pastor, must not only carry out his professional functions objectively, but at all times and seasons he must play the role of pastor in a flawless manner. Society demands this as a kind of security ... It is therefore not surprising that everyone who wants to be successful has to take these expectations into account.

The construction of a collectively suitable *persona* means a very great concession to the outer world. It is a real self-sacrifice which directly

forces the ego into an identification with the *persona,* so that there are
people who actually believe themselves to be what they present to the
public view.... These identifications with the social role are a very fruitful
source of neuroses. *A man cannot get rid of himself in favor of an artificial
personality without punishment.* The mere attempt to do so releases, in
all the ordinary cases, unconscious reactions in the form of moods, affects,
fears, compulsive ideas, feelings, vices, etc. (White, 1948, p. 166; my
emphasis).

The neurotic is caught up in attempting to be something he is
not, in line with social expectations. He may be the individual who
changes his name to ward off negative social valuations, only to
find that this is not the answer to the problem of valuing himself
for what he is, and his cultural subgroup for what it is. Thus, a
report in *Commentary* (Kugelmass, 1952) notes that in an investigation of a group of Jewish subjects who had changed their last
names because they felt their names made them or their children
especially subject to prejudice, it was found that not one of them
was happy with the change. This finding may be contrasted with
the change of name which emphasizes or asserts one's identity, as
in taking a Hebrew name.

Schizophrenia

Some kinds of schizophrenic breakdown also lend themselves to
an interpretation in terms of the theory and concepts offered here.
On the basis of a study of 36 male and 17 female schizophrenics,
Weinberg has offered such a theory:

First, these schizophrenics were not what would be called shut-in "seclu-
sive" types. But some were isolated from the persons or from the cultural
skills in those areas of behavior in which their conflicts were to become
most intense and threatening. Second, they participated in intimate
groups until the very onset of the disorder. Third, it was not the isolation
but the meaning and reaction to isolation that bore most significantly upon
eventual schizophrenic behavior. This became especially pertinent in the
disruption of such intimate contacts as courtship and marital relations.
Thus, personal isolation becomes significant only as it reflects upon the
person's irreconcilable and unbearable conflicts, and it cannot be understood without these conflicts.

These conflicts are so unbearable because they are so self-involving.
The schizophrenic regards himself as a failure and/or completely loses
confidence in his ability to manipulate his environment. The eleven subjects who attempted suicide exemplified this effort to destroy a reproach-
ful self-image. The others who acted out against their relatives, spouses
and other persons regarded this behavior as a random bid for regaining

their self-esteem. The crucial forms of isolation among schizophrenics emerge from the following personal experiences: 1) they reject the self-image but strive for self-acceptance and social acceptance; 2) they are unable to communicate their conflicts to other persons, or do not have accessible persons to whom they can communicate their conflicts; and 3) they resort to withdrawal as a medium of self-protection. This withdrawing process is not merely a segregating process, but rather a disruption in role-taking. For the disruption in role-taking has a protective effect upon the schizophrenic insofar as it spares him from accepting the evaluations of others and looking back at himself. This disruption in role-taking and self-reference is basic to the subsequent disorientations and false extrapolations which Devereau has emphasized, for disoriented behavior means that the psychotic is unable to shift his perspective and share the perspectives of others.

Though chronic schizophrenics also tend to respond in this way, their reactions to unacceptable self-evaluations are not as intense as among transient schizophrenics. The chronic schizophrenics seem more likely to accept the lowered verdict of themselves and to readjust to it. The transient schizophrenics do not accept this lowered self-verdict but fight it, and in this fight are more likely to achieve the kind of personal reorientation which makes the disorder relatively brief and improvement come relatively quick (Weinberg, 1955, pp. 256-257).

Thus, the dynamics for each of these different kinds of behavior may be understood in terms of the concepts and theory suggested by the study of first names.

IMPLICATIONS FOR RESEARCH AND PRACTICE

The methodology used here in an investigation of first names may also be applied to such aspects of the self-concept as religion, physical appearance, occupation, education, color, social class, and so forth, in an exploration of the relations between self-identity, self-acceptance, and individual and group attitudes toward significant aspects of the self. How are any of these singly or in combination related to self-identity and self-acceptance? A refined questionnaire around the first and other names might form a simple but useful instrument for investigating attitudes toward the self.

The formation and fostering of groups in which individuals will find a sense of belonging and a positive valuation of their own characteristics are needed. The insights stemming from such groups as Alcoholics Anonymous and Synanon and from the therapeutic community have something to offer here. So would a study of the kinds of steps minority members have taken to build and maintain their own self-esteem. Aichhorn (1951) has described how even extremely aggressive delinquents can, under the right conditions and in due time, form a very cohesive group. Kevin (1963) has also described how a group consultation method can be used to establish a group program in a welfare department.

In connection with the investigation of such groups, a study of the "unintegrated" or "peripheral" member or members is important. Weinberg (1955) has noted that schizophrenics tend to be peripheral to their families; French and his associates (1962) have noted that in an industrial setting, members occupying peripheral positions tend to have lower self-esteem. The contributions of the group-dynamics investigators with respect to leadership, structure, process, cohesiveness, planned change, and other aspects of group functioning are relevant here.

It may be suggested that there is need for a way to investigate clusters of groups and to study how to strengthen them. Studies of cohesive families have shown that they are to be found in a network of cohesive families (Zimmerman & Cervantes, 1960). And as we look beyond the individual group to the interrelations among different groups, we move toward another way of approaching the total community.

ISSUES CONCERNING RESEARCH IN COMMUNITY PSYCHOLOGY

In conclusion, I should like to raise two issues with respect to the research and theory reported in this chapter: (1) the need for a central value base, and (2) the wider context in which research in community psychology and community mental health is carried out.

Does research in community psychology, which is more directly concerned with the understanding and resolution of social, community, and individual problems, have to be more explicit about its value base than does laboratory-oriented social psychology? Is "growth" such a concept, and is self-acceptance (a variable used in this investigation) one of the significant aspects of growth?

MacKinnon and Maslow called for such an orientation almost two decades ago, when they wrote:

Most important for motivation and value-theory is the introduction of a positive force to supplement the Freudian pessimism and the neo-behavioristic relativism which in general assumes that the organism is ultimately motivated by avoidance of punishment, the relief of tension, and the seeking for a few physiological pleasures, e.g., food, sex, etc., and by whatever can be learned on this basis....

What such a positive concept can do for psychology is seen in the numerous writings of [Carl] Rogers ... and his students, in which the concept of "growth" (indistinguishable from self-actualization) assumes more and more a central and essential role. This can be equally so for a psychological theory of democracy, of interpersonal relations, of social improvement, of cross-cultural comparison, and of a scientific system of values. With its aid there is no reason why cognition, conation, and affection should not be tied together once again, i.e., the contrast between individual and social, between selfish and altruistic, between instinctive and rational, and many other such false dichotomies can be resolved (MacKinnon & Maslow, 1951, p. 646).

As regards the wider context of research in community psychology and community mental health, this study has explored interrelations between social valuation and self-valuation—one significant aspect of the relations between community and individual. In community psychology the concern is with the whole complex of institutions, laws, agencies, ways of delivering service, definitions of deviancy and illness, power structures, and so on, which are related to these social valuations, and actions or behaviors toward "deviant" and nondeviant individuals. It is, of course, the wider public which carries the ultimate responsibility for supporting or changing these definitions and institutions.

Research problems and research methodology in community psychology need to be redefined and designed to take this broader picture into account. Even as we look for individual growth, we look for growth (change) in laws, agencies, institutions. For the laws may be intimately related to the resolution of a major problem such as alcoholism—as is suggested, for example, by Sanford in Chapter 9 of this volume. Research on a particular problem area is therefore concerned not only with a narrowly defined approach, as in the evaluation of a particular program or assessment of mental illness in a particular community, but should take this wider context into account, as, for example, with historical and cross-cultural investigations. Researchers will then be in a better position to assess and interpret their findings, with respect to any particular problem, to the wider community which provides the base and sanction for further action.

REFERENCES

Adelson, D. An exploratory study of stereotypy: impressions of personality formed from mere knowledge of personal names. Unpublished paper, 1953.

Adelson, D. Some aspects of value conflict under extreme conditions. *Psychiat.*, 1962, **25** (3), 273-279.

Adelson, D. Attitudes toward first names. *Proc. First International Congress of Social Psychiatry*, London, Special Edition No. 1, August, 1964. Based on a dissertation submitted in partial fulfillment of the requirements for the degree of Doctor of Philosophy under the Joint Committee on Graduate Instruction, Columbia Univer. (a)

Adelson, D. Social factors in the placement of the chronic schizophrenic patient. *Amer. J. Psychiat.*, 1964, **121** (1), 61-64. (b)

Aichhorn, A. *Wayward youth.* (Rev. ed.) London: Imago Pub. Co., 1951.

Angyal, A. *Foundations for a science of personality.* New York: Commonwealth Fund, 1941.

Asch, S. E. Effects of group pressure upon the modification and distortion of judgments. In D. Cartwright & A. Zander (Eds.), *Group dynamics: research and theory.* Evanston, Ill.: Row, Peterson, 1960.

Bennis, W. G., & Shepard, H. A theory of group development. In W. G. Bennis, K. D. Benne, & R. Chin (Eds.), *The planning of change: readings in the applied behavioral sciences.* New York: Holt, Rinehart & Winston, 1961.

Berger, E. M. The relation between expressed acceptance of self and expressed acceptance of others. *J. abnorm. soc. Psychol.*, 1952, **47**, 778-782.

Bugental, J. F. T., & Zelen, S. F. Investigations into the self concept. *J. Pers.*, 1950, **18**, 483-498.

Clark, K. B., & Clark, M. P. Racial identification and preference in Negro children. In T. M. Newcomb & R. L. Hartley (Eds.), *Readings in social psychology.* New York: Holt, 1947.

Cohen, A. K. Delinquent boys: the culture of the group. As interpreted in C. Selltiz, M. Jahoda, M. Deutsch, & S. W. Cook, *Research methods in social relations.* (Rev. ed.) New York: Holt, 1959.

Crutchfield, R. Conformity and character. *Amer. Psychologist,* 1955, **10**, 191-198.

Cumming, E., & Cumming, J. *Closed ranks: an experiment in mental health education.* Cambridge: Harvard Univer. Press, 1957.

Duss, Louisa. Fonction psychologique du nom proper dans la reconstruction de la personalite d'une schizophrene. *J. Psychol. norm. path.*, 1946, **39**, 350-366.

French, J. P. R., Kahn, R. L., & Mann, F. C. Work, health and satisfaction. *J. soc. Issues,* 1962, **18** (3), 1-129.

Hildreth, Gertrude. Development of sequences in name writing. *Child Develpm.*, 1936, **7**, 291-303.

Jahoda, M. A note on Ashanti names and their relationship to personality. *Brit. J. Psychol.*, 1954, **45**, 190-195.

Jahoda, M. *Current concepts of positive mental health.* New York: Basic Books, 1958.

James, W. *Psychology* (Briefer Course). Cleveland: World Pub., 1948.

Kevin, D. An analysis of the group consultation method in the establishment of a group program in a welfare department. Unpublished manuscript, 1963.

Kugelmass, J. A. Name changing—and what it gets you. *Commentary*, 1952, **14**, 145-150.

Leighton, A. *The governing of men.* Princeton, N.J.: Princeton Univer. Press, 1945.

Lewin, K. *Resolving social conflicts.* New York: Harper, 1948.

Levy, D. M. *Maternal overprotection.* New York: Columbia Univer. Press, 1943.

MacKinnon, D. W., & Maslow, A. H. Personality. In H. Helson (Ed.), *Theoretical foundations of psychology.* New York: Van Nostrand, 1951.

Mead, G. H. *Mind, self and society from the standpoint of a social behaviorist.* Chicago: Univer. of Chicago Press, 1934.

Mullahy, P. *Oedipus myth and complex: a review of psychoanalytic theory.* New York: Grove, 1955.

Murphy, G. *Personality: a personal approach to origins and structure.* New York: Harper, 1947.

Sampson, H., Messinger, S. L., & Towne, R. D. *Schizophrenic women: studies in marital crisis.* New York: Atherton, 1964.

Schoenfeld, N. An experimental study of some problems relating to stereotypes. *Arch. Psychol.*, 1942, No. 270, p. 55.

Slavson, S. R. *An introduction to group therapy.* New York: Commonwealth Fund, 1943.

Weinberg, S. K. A sociological analysis of a schizophrenic type. In A. M. Rose (Ed.), *Mental health and mental disorder.* New York: Norton, 1955.

White, R. W. *The abnormal personality: a textbook.* New York: Ronald, 1948.

Zimmerman, C. C., & Cervantes, L. F. *Successful American families.* New York: Pageant Press, 1960.

CHAPTER 8

Toward an Ecological Conception of Preventive Interventions

James G. Kelly

The work described in this paper on natural environments is designed as an aid in conceptualizing preventive interventions. Primary interest is in such questions as: (1) What types of psychological treatments are relevant for social settings? (2) What are the effects of such treatments upon the behavior of participants in social settings? (3) What change in organizational functions will emerge as a result of interventions?

From the writer's experience in developing preventive services in different parts of the country, the effects of geographical and cultural diversity in limiting or accelerating the development of community services have been clearly observed. The attempt in this paper is to contribute a conception of preventive interventions by a study of natural environments.

More specifically, an emerging ecological thesis will be presented by illustrating the kinds of integrative tasks involved in this research program. As an introduction for this thesis, four principles from field biology will be presented to provide the context for the discussion of the research program and its implications for preventive services.

ECOLOGICAL ANALOGIES

Elsewhere the writer has presented a case for the ecological analogy, both for studying social environments and for changing

This article is Chapter 6 of *Research Contributions from Psychology to Community Mental Health*, edited by Dr. Jerry W. Carter, Jr., published in 1969 by Behavioral Publications, Inc., 2852 Broadway, New York, N.Y.

them (Kelly, 1966a, 1966b, 1967). The premise for this analogy is relevant for studying the expression of effectiveness in varied environments, e.g., this axiom states that functions of individuals and organizations are interdependent.

The translations of this particular ecological analogy affirms that as the structure and functions of social units vary, modes of dealing with disruptive events also shift, with a corresponding variation in the behavior of individuals who perform adaptive and maladaptive roles in the specific society. Interrelationships between the functions of social units and the participation of individual members then become a primary focus for designing programs of interventions where the intervention rearranges the interrelationships or couplings between individual behavior and social functions as much as it alters the behavior of one social unit or the expressive behavior of any one member of the society. The work of the writer includes such specific variables as: (a) individual preferences for dealing with environments (coping styles); (b) the development of role requirements for social settings (adaptive role functions); (c) the type and range of units for social interaction that are characteristic of specific environments (social settings); and (d) the structural properties of the environment, such as rate of population exchange. The development of a conception for these four types of variables can then lead to the design of interventions based upon knowledge for topics like: (1) What styles of coping behavior are correlated with effective performance in varied environments? (2) How are adaptive roles distributed in different environments? (3) How do changes in the structures of social environments effect changes in social functions? The primary integrative and conceptual task is to specify how these four types of variables are interrelated.

Before discussing the interrelationships for these variables in more detail, a few comments are in order about ecological analogies. Ecology, with its concern with the relationship of organisms or groups of organisms with their environment, historically has been a multidisciplinary enterprise. Smith (1966) cites Macfadyen (1957), who has made the following observations about the scope of ecology:

The ecologist is something of a chartered libertine. He roams at will over the legitimate preserves of the plant and animal biologist, the taxonomist, the physiologist, the behaviorist, the meteorologist, the geologist, the physicist, the chemist, and even the sociologist; he poaches from all these and from other established and respected disciplines. It is indeed a major problem for the ecologist, in his interest, to set bounds to his divagations. (Smith, 1966, p. 5)

In spite of the breadth of the field and the number of relevant disciplines involved, there are some principles that have an empirical basis in field biology and that offer a point of departure for the study of social environments.

Principle I: Functions within a Social Unit Are Interdependent (The Ecosystem Principle)

One of the primary analytic terms in field biology is the concept of the ecosystem, the interdependence of living and nonliving elements. This term uniquely defines the emergence of ecology as an identifiable point of view. A brief summary of the principle can be stated like this:

... a naturally occurring assemblage of plants and animals that live in the same environment, are mutually sustaining and interdependent, and are constantly fixing, utilizing and dissipating energy. The interacting populations are characterized by constant death and replacement and usually by immigration and emigration of individuals. The populations are always fluctuating with seasonal and environmental changes. The community depends upon and is influenced by the habitat, the specific set of conditions that surround the organisms, such as sunlight, soil, mineral elements, moisture, temperature, and topography. The biotic (living) and the abiotic (nonliving) interact, thus creating an ecological system or *ecosystem*. (Smith, 1966, pp. 12-13)

This principle of interdependence or reciprocity between structures and functions is one of the axioms for the ecologist (see Watt, 1967, as a very recent example). One implication of the knowledge generated from ecosystem studies of the natural habitat is the awareness that organisms depend not only upon food sources but also directly or indirectly upon one another for their well-being and existence.

The translation of this axiom for a study of social environments presents difficulties since psychologists do not often view the coupling of structure and function as the focus for theory construction. More often we select one aspect of social structure, i.e., social class, and study its effects upon individuals who vary along certain dimensions, such as response to psychotherapy. We also will select individuals, such as persons who vary in their attitudes (dogmatism) and identify how the function in an organization (resist change). Both of these prototypic methods do not, however, usually include hypotheses or inferences that focus on a conception of cause and effect as one of interdependence between social class and response to therapy or dogmatism and organizational participation.

Roger Barker's work and that of his students and colleagues is a distinguished and notable exception in psychology not only for the methodological contributions in defining the social setting, but for their efforts to identify the effects of such variables as size and physical distance upon the behavior of participants (Barker, 1960, 1964, 1965). However, as Sommer's (1967) recent review indicates, much of this type of work and other research on the ecology of group behavior is taxonomic or descriptive and is not concerned with explicating the social processes that mediate between such variables as size or density of a setting and the behavior of individual group members.

The translation of the ecological analogy for designing preventive services requires a definition of the functions of a society in conjunction with a view of those persons who are unique in performing or not performing adaptive functions. The creation of hypotheses for such interdependence should be derived from a motivational theory that is ecological. For the present work I am asking: What social functions are generated for high school students attending a school with a high rate of exchange? How do students attending a school with high preferences for exploration fulfill or take part in such functions? What are the effects of such interrelationships for the performance of adaptive and maladaptive behavior of the organization and its members?

Principle II: The Cycling of Resources

This principle as it applies to field biology is a corollary of the first principle and is a direct derivation from the laws of thermodynamics. The first law of thermodynamics is often translated to mean that energy is transferred, neither created nor destroyed, while the second law of thermodynamics states that the transformation of energy assumes a form that cannot be passed on any further. In biology this principle is expressed by methods for defining how energy is transferred from one organism to another and how a large part of that energy is degraded as heat with the remainder stored as living tissue. An example of the cycling of resources in animal ecology is the food chain. Marsh vegetation is eaten by the grasshopper, the grasshopper is consumed by the shrew, the shrew, by the marsh hawk or the owl, with the effect that no organism lives wholly on another but resources are shared. From this principle, measurement of the production of energy in different plant or animal communities has been attempted in order to specify how net and gross production varies among plant communities and to determine the efficiency of production of communities—the useful output of energy in relation to input.

The translation of this principle of energy transfer to the measurement of social environments is undeveloped. Except for contemporary organizational psychologists such as Katz and Kahn (1966) and a few of the studies cited by Pugh's (1966) recent review, an equivalent concept is not developed. For the development of interventions, assessment of the procedures for utilizing resources is essential in order to clarify how skills are distributed in an organization and how an organization shares competences.

Viewing social environments in this light does make it possible to view the developmental history of an organization in terms of its management of resources. Katz and Kahn (1966, p. 161), for instance, present as one approach for defining organizational efficiency the ratio of energic output to energic input. They attempt to conceive how much input to an organization emerges as product and how much is absorbed by the system.

One implication of this principle for my own work is a study of the effects of population exchange of high school students upon the development and absorption of informal leaders. My guess is that high exchange environments make more efficient use of resources than low exchange environments. One of the predicted adaptive responses an organization can make to a high rate of population exchange is an unplanned-for increase in utilizing rare resources.

Principle III: The Environment Affects Styles of Adaptation

This principle derives from Von Lubig's law of minimum and Shelford's later modification of the law of tolerance (Smith, 1966, p. 60). The modern derivation of these laws states that the availability of nutrient substances affects the presence of an organism. The empirical research on this law has demonstrated that an organism that exhibits a wide range of tolerance for all environmental influences will be widely distributed in multiple and contrasting settings (Ardrey, 1966; Smith, 1966). Current research in field biology concerned with this principle is focusing upon a re-examination of evolutionary theory, and is leading to restatements of natural selection (Simpson, 1967; Williams, 1966).

Levins, in discussing the context for the construction of model building on biology, concludes that work on the joint evolution of habitat selection and niche breadth, on the role of productivity of biotic environments and on food-getting procedures, all converge in supporting the theorem that environmental uncertainty (randomness) leads to increased niche breadth while unchanging environments lead to specialization of members (Levins, 1966, pp. 426-427). Such work as Levins' and that of Lewontin (1938), who has defined adaptive behavior as the relative diversity of environments in which a unit of evolution can survive and reproduce, provides a provocative set of questions for specifying the form of adaptations for varied social environments.

Principle IV: The Succession Principle: The Evolution of Natural Communities

The principle of succession is characterized by progressive changes in species structure, in organic structure, and in energy flow. In field biology, the principle assumes that there is a gradual and continuous replacement of one kind of plant and animal by another, until the community itself is replaced by another that is more complex. This principle focuses on those factors that contribute toward progressive change in species structure and the changes in the flow of energy distribution and community production. This process in biology assumes that as organisms exploit the environment, their own activities make a habitat unfavorable for their own survival. But in doing so, they create an environment for a different group of organisms, with an equilibrium or steady state with the environment that is more or less achieved for a limited period of time. As natural environments receive greater and greater modification, the succession process is altered, affecting the composition and even the functions of communities. This phenomenon is the subject for much of the theory, research, and contemporary work in conservation. As Smith summarizes:

To provide food for himself, man has cleared away natural vegetation and replaced it with simple, highly artificial communities of cultivated species, adapted to grow on disturbed sites. This has brought about an explosion of insect pests and accelerated erosion of unprotected soil. Nowhere is land change more complete than in industrial and urban areas, a climax type of human succession. Natural communities are completely destroyed and replaced by the concrete, asphalt, and steel of cities, highways, and dams. And the process is accompanied by air and water pollution from industrial and human wastes. Most communities exist only through man's continued, deliberate interference, usually motivated by economic interests. In these "economic climaxes," the animals and plants present either are desired by man or are adaptable to existing conditions. (Smith, 1966, p. 155)

This principle of succession is particularly relevant for studying social environments, for the principle defines a time perspective for the organization, and alerts the investigator to assess and define the systemic change already present in the organization prior to any proposed intervention. It is also an aid in drawing implications for the relevance of the adaptive effects of specific coping processes. To the extent that a high exchange environment is approaching constancy or a low exchange environment is unsettling, changes will be expected in how persons who vary in their coping preferences assume adaptive or maladaptive roles. For example, persons with high preferences for exploration will be able to assume more adaptive roles as the environment becomes less constant and more fluid.

SUMMARY OF A RESEARCH EXAMPLE: A STUDY OF ADAPTIVE BEHAVIOR IN VARIED HIGH SCHOOL ENVIRONMENTS

These four principles have provided the context for the development of a conception of the coupling process between individuals and organizations and provides a dynamic understanding of the role of individuals in large organizations, and the relative levels of ineffectiveness and effectiveness that are specific for particular environments.

The major work is a study of teenagers' preferences for coping with their high school environment. The specific coping style selected for study is exploratory behavior. Exploration is defined as preferences for trying out alternative behaviors and sampling diverse social situations in the high schools. A 30-item paper and pencil questionnaire and the description of preliminary work carried out in two high schools in Columbus, Ohio, has been described previously (Kelly, 1966a, 1967).

The current research is planned as a longitudinal study of four cohorts of male high school students, who vary in their preferences for exploratory behavior, and who are attending high school environments that contrast in the number of students who enter and leave during a school year. Two high schools of equal size have been selected from a suburban area of Detroit. One of these high schools has an exchange rate of students that is 22 per cent, while the other school has an exchange rate that is only 6 per cent. Two other high schools of equal size and of equal demographic characteristics have been selected in the inner city of Detroit. One of these inner city schools has an exchange rate of 50 per cent of its students, while the second school has an exchange rate of 15 per cent.

Population exchange has been selected as the main independent variable for defining the social environments of these two schools, because of the premise that rate of population turnover has predictable effects not only upon the social functions in these two environments but also upon the coping preferences of the students. For example, one hypothesis states that students who have high preferences for exploration will have a high probability of emerging as adaptive members in a fluid environment but will develop maladaptive roles in a constant environment. Male high school students who are low explorers will have a contrasting adaptive history and are predicted to emerge as effective members in a constant society, but are more likely to assume maladaptive behaviors in a fluid environment. The research will involve studies of the peer society, and faculty-student relations as well as naturalistic observations of relevant social settings in order to present a comprehensive view of the context of exploratory behavior.*

My interest in developing principles of intervention from an ecological conception of adaptation is derived from the conviction that most programs of individual or organizational change focus on either organizational behavior or the activities of specific individu-

---

*See Orth, 1962; Mechanic, 1962; and Becker *et al.*, 1961, as examples of studies of coping responses to social environments; Lazarus (1966) presents a review of the recent experimental and theoretical literature on the topic. Klein and Lindemann (1961) and Caplan (1964) provide excellent conceptions for preventive services.

als, with only slight consideration of the interdependence of individuals *and* the organization or the benefits and costs of any intervention for individuals *or* organizations. What this research is aimed toward is the creation of empirical knowledge of the interdependence of societies and their members. It is my belief that without knowledge of the process of adaptation to varied environments, it will not be possible to evolve a science of interventions. The remainder of these comments will focus upon some ideas about how the primary variables of the research can be defined in an a priori fashion as interdependent.

Individual Coping Styles (Exploratory Behavior)

One of the interpretations of an ecological analogy is that the dominance of certain behaviors will be specific for social settings (Smith, 1966; Kelly, 1967). As has been mentioned, the general class of environments studied is high schools. It has been assumed that the behavior of students in the high school will affect their behavior when they are not in school. It was also thought that life in the high school would have observable effects upon the socialization process of the adolescent, a critical data source for planning and evaluating interventions.

In concluding an analysis of sources of behavioral variance dealing with anxiousness, Endler and Hunt (1966, p. 345) conclude:

The fact that interactions contribute approximately a third of the variance implies that personality descriptions can be improved by describing people in terms of responses they manifest in various kinds of situations.

The writer, in taking this mandate seriously, has asserted that male high school students who are high in their preferences for exploration are predicted to undertake more adaptive roles in a high turnover environment than in another. The research also is aimed to define the type of roles students will perform in the school setting as well as the type of behavior they will manifest in varied social settings.

Exploratory behavior has been identified as having different effects for the expression of social competence in varied environments. The term refers to preferences for participation in varied social settings and an attraction for novel or unique social situations, and is currently measured by a 30-item paper and pencil questionnaire with items such as "I like staying home and keeping friendships with people I've known a long time," and "I don't like it when a special TV program takes the place of the one I usually watch." On the basis of pilot studies, these scales have been found to be uncorrelated with social desirability, independent of measures of other coping styles, and positively related to Rotter's measure of internal-external control (Kelly, 1966; Rotter, 1966).

Preliminary findings have suggested partial validity since male high school students who were defined as high explorers had a higher probability of being nominated as deviant members in a high school with little population exchange than did students who preferred low exploratory activities (Kelly, 1966). It is hoped that one of the by-products of this approach to construct validation is to specify the diverse conditions for expression of exploratory behavior.

Conception of Adaptive Roles

The ecological analogy also assumes that as environments vary so do the adaptive and maladaptive behaviors they generate. Defining adaptive roles for a particular social environment highlights two complementary issues: the relationship between the social settings and the type of adaptive behaviors that develop in such settings, and the second issue is the type of personality variables that are correlated with adaptive roles. For the present work, the prediction is that persons who prefer one coping style will fulfill comparable organizational requirements. For example, persons who have expressed a preference for high exploratory behavior will emerge as effective in performing the following activities: (a) assessment of alternatives for solving organizational problems (analysis); (b) proposing recommendations for organizational change (criticism); (c) defining new activities, new norms or new modes of social control for that environment (planning); (d) identifying relationships of the present environment with other resources (scouting). Adaptive roles that the person with high preferences for exploration is not likely to value or take part in are (a) implementing a solution for one specific activity or event (execution); (b) monitoring current activities, norms, or modes of social control for the organization (surveillance); (c) assessing the members' responses to the current environment (facilitation); (d) identifying obstacles limiting operation of the organization (confirmation).

While both kinds of behaviors are identified as essential for every organization, it is assumed that environments with a high exchange of members will generally reward and value the first set of adaptive roles rather than the second set. This latter set of roles will be viewed as more congruent for organizations with little exchange in their membership. It is expected that there is a selective process operating for each of these environments whereby high explorers will adopt the first set of roles and not the others. Postulating this distinction between differences in individuals and variations in organizations hopefully will generate data to clarify not only the varieties of adaptive roles within an organization but also the relationship between personality and organizational variables.

Social Setting

The measurement of social settings, the spatial locations for social interaction within environments, provides a definition for those aspects of the structure of the environment that are related directly to the expression of adaptive roles as just described. Again the interdependence of individual behavior and organizational roles is linked with the functional taxonomy of the organization and its environmental form.

Where 50 per cent of the members of an environment come and go during any period of the life cycle of the organization, there will be greater quantity of social settings than are expected for an environment in which only a small percentage of its members are new. The value attached to participation in social settings in the high-exchange environment is also expected to vary considerably over time, so that new settings will arise, have a short life history, and then be replaced by new modes of action correlating with the changing standards for that environment. Conversely, social participation and social interaction in the constant environment are predicted to have a smaller number of settings that are not expected to change over time. These predictions for the effects of population exchange complement Barker's findings on the effects of school size on social settings (Barker, 1964). He found that although there was a greater number of settings in the large schools, more students took part in the affairs of the small schools. The student body in the large high schools did not participate in the larger number of available activities. The present work suggests that a fluid environment can compensate for the negative effects of large size by generating new settings as a consequence of population exchange.

Another prediction for the effects of rate of population exchange upon the functions of social settings is the level of the formality of the settings. The social process in a high-exchange environment is as likely to occur in informal social interactions, on playgrounds, at football games, in the cafeteria, or at the favorite pizzeria. The settings at the constant school are expected to be almost identical with the formal settings such as the classroom, assembly halls, study halls, and at the meeting places for extracurricular activities. There are also expected to be differences for behavior expressed in school settings and those outside of school. For the fluid environment, what one does in school and on school property will be equivalent to the same wide range of behavior expressed off school grounds. An analysis of the social settings at the constant school will present more dichotomous behavior. More students will be doing the same things in the same way over a long period of time in school, yet will be doing quite different things in their leisure activity. It is a guess that the almost complete predictability of the constant environment for the students will function as a motivator for seeking uniqueness in new environments.

Wheeler (Brim & Wheeler, 1966, p. 78) has suggested two concepts for studying the structures of socialization settings that are also apt for making additional predictions for social participation in these contrasting environments. In discussing the idea that authorities in organizations vary in their response to recruits, he states that in *homogenizing settings* there is a tendency to reduce the relevance of prior experience for present adjustment. In *differentiating settings,* there may be an urging of recruits to give expression to the different backgrounds and interests they bring into the organization. In the present example, fluid environments would be expected to have more differentiating settings, while constant environments would be predicted to generate more homogenizing settings. On the basis of preliminary findings of organizational responses to newcomers in two Columbus, Ohio, high schools, this is the case (Kelly, 1966, 1967). New students at the fluid environment were actively welcomed, were informed of both acceptable and unacceptable activities going on at the school and were given a mandate, "Try us out." New students not only perceived that the total resources of the school were available to them but they reported that their previous activities and experiences were utilized. New students at the constant school seemed compelled to make the first move and were judged, studied, and categorized according to the existing social order before any social relationships began and then only with persons in equivalent status positions.

Effects of Environmental Exchange

Before discussing the nature of the integrative tasks for this work and the implications for designing interventions, brief comments will be made on the predictive power of population exchange as a unit in the ecological chain. It is assumed that this variable will affect not only the number and range of social settings but the generation of adaptive roles and the socialization for exploratory behavior. This particular ecological variable was selected for study not only for its intrinsic value but because of the number of parallel predictions that can be generated for the effects of this type of environment upon a range of plant and animal populations (Smith, 1966; Levins, 1967). The other primary reason for the selection of this particular variable is that it should be possible to document the simultaneous effects of how individuals (explorers) respond (take adaptive roles) in varied environments and how organizations respond (generate social settings and adaptive roles) to varied rates of immigration and emigration.

INTEGRATIVE TASKS

Interdependence of Variables

This work requires at least three distinct integrative tasks. One is the conceptual integration of the interdependence of variables, which has been mentioned. A second is the integration of methods and the third is the integration of theory with practice.

Specifying the environmental conditions for various forms of behavior can provide two sources of data for defining mental health. One is the effects of an organization upon specific coping styles, in persons performing specific adaptive roles. The second is an analysis of the consequences of adaptive performance in one organization as it relates for membership in a new organization. An adaptive member of a fluid environment may learn the rudiments of innovative behavior, but if faced with physical relocation may perceive himself to be in crisis. The adaptive member of a constant environment may learn a set of specialized roles and the rudiments of citizenship, but react in a maladaptive fashion in an organization when he is relocated or when his environment undergoes rapid changes. The provision for a cohort design in each of the selected high schools will be created to assess the profits and costs for high and low explorers who are living in these contrasting environments. If this kind of integration can be made, it will help to define the context for generating varieties of "healthy" behavior.

Utility of Multiple Methods

In the preliminary work, two methods have been used, a paper and pencil questionnaire to assess coping preferences, and naturalistic observations to document the type and range of social settings within each school. The next phase of this work will include additional methods to reduce the effects of method variance, and to represent the intricacies of the environment. Survey instruments will be created to assess the perceptions of the students and faculty regarding the normative rules within the school and the mode of faculty-student relations. Intensive case studies will also be conducted with a sample of high and low explorers in order to provide complementary information regarding their perceptions of the environment and their views of the socialization process.

One of the major methodological assignments is to create data collection procedures so that an estimate can be made of the research process on the natural life of the environment. On the basis of preliminary work, it was found that observing hallways in the fluid school seemed to have no noticeable effect on the students' behavior. The same observers, however, in a constant school were perceived by both faculty and students as an intrusion. For the present work we will recruit high school students from the host school to carry out observations in the schools and to employ video tape recordings to supplement these personal observations. Also, we will be responsive to document the effects of naturally occurring crises in the local communities and schools. The diversity of methods to be employed is intended to increase the precision of assessing the school societies as they respond to unplanned events.

Theory and Practice

The integrative task of linking theory to practice is provocative since it focuses on the utility of knowledge. The objective of this work is to contribute basic knowledge about relationships between social structures and individual coping styles in order to establish an ecological basis for deducing preventive services. One axiom of the ecologist is that an intervention in one part of the organization will affect the total organization. An ecological orientation is particularly apt for most community mental health services, because not only are preventive services usually imposed or added onto an ongoing program, but by nature of preventive work, multiple agencies and organizations are usually involved as participants if not consumers.

Geertz (1963) reports an example, attributed to the ecologist Clarke (Clarke, 1954), that illustrates an ecological chain. Clarke tells of ranchers,

... who disturbed by losses of young sheep to coyotes, slaughtered, through collective effort, nearly all coyotes in the immediate area. Following the removal of coyotes, the rabbits, field mice, and other small rodents, upon whom the coyotes had previously preyed, multiplied rapidly and made serious inroads on the grass of the pastures. When this was realized, the sheep men ceased to kill coyotes and instituted an elaborate program for the poisoning of rodents. The coyotes filtered in from the surrounding areas, but finding their natural rodent food now scarce, were forced to turn with even greater intensity to the young sheep as their only available source of food (pp. 4-5).

While there is no intent here to equate mental health professionals with these ranchers, mental health programs do not always anticipate any adverse effects of their interventions for the resources of the community or the functions of key persons. A more prevalent view is to alter overt behavior with minimal assessment of organizational or personal side effects. One ethic for the ecologist is to assess the host organization in order to anticipate the effects of the intervention upon the functions of the organization.

Referring to constant and fluid environments as examples, it is predicted that reports of mental health problems in a constant environment will be quite different from the reported concerns from the fluid environment. In the constant environment with its value for absorption for its members, persons of this setting will be expected to ask for help for those persons who "criticize," who question normative structures, or who may "agitate for change." The treatment fantasies of the faculty will be to "fit" students in or exclude them. Faculties from the fluid schools who are oriented by necessity to develop and actualize their members will tend to see anybody who prefers "direction" as a person in "crisis" and will want advice from the consultant on how to motivate him.

These predictions about the effects of living in these two diverse environments and the generation of maladaptive behaviors lead to quite different proposals for interventions. For the remainder of these comments examples of interventions considered relevant for these two contrasting environments will be presented.

CONTRASTING INTERVENTIONS

A change program for the fluid environment would be designed as a program aimed to improve the socialization for the students of the high school.* The change programs for the constant high school would be focused on the adult faculty and administration, with less attention to the student body. The purposes of these interventions are different, as are the methods and style of the change agents and the bases for evaluating program success.

Socialization Aid for a Fluid Environment

A tentative intervention for this setting is to supplement existing informal and formal social processes and promote the identity development of the students. Older high school students, high school graduates, and a variety of formal and informal community resources could be involved to strengthen the existing life of the high-exchange environment, without limiting the open-ended quality of the environment or creating new organizational structures. Change agents working in this program would be trying to facilitate the operation of the fluctuating activities of these multiple social units. For example, simultaneous programs, such as car maintenance, athletic skill development, vocational training, educational enrichment, could be interventions for school environments that are fluid and serving lower-class populations. Equivalent socialization programs relating to leisure-time activities, such as sailing clubs, as well as courses and seminars relating to personal development, would be the suggested content for stu-

*See H. Bredemeier (1964) for a comprehensive socialization program that does not take into account diverse environments.

dents from fluid schools serving a higher socioeconomic class. Tutorial programs with informal supervision by peers and adults would characterize the relationship of the change agents and the clients in both types of fluid schools.

The time periods needed for developing these contrasting programs would vary as well. For instance, there would be a short period of preparation and a longer period of implementation for the fluid high school. Because this type of school is expected to define change as a way of life, the school authorities and students will not require long periods of orientation, warm-ups, clarification, and rationales; their thirst for action will lead to instant programming. To refine the intervention and to enable the program to become an integral part of the total society, a longer period of time would be required. This difference in the metric of the intervention is a consequence not only of the students' and faculty's unfamiliarity in coping with intact organizational structures but also because of the time required to establish functional communication for all the diverse and scattered units of this changing environment.

An evaluation of the interventions for this type of environment could be measured by phrasing questions such as: Will a person with preferences for exploration be able to develop a self-perception and self-esteem as a risk-taker? Does he emerge with a self-perception of a more integrated individual? If the interventions have been effective the high explorer, in addition to surviving in a chaotic society, should be able to differentiate himself in that society.

Faculty Development for a Constant Environment

This type of social environment could receive an equal number of services but in this case they are faculty-oriented, to allow the faculty to consider the expected personal costs for those students attending such an environment. The interventions could be provided by a variety of professional persons and could include various forms of human relations training and consultative services, including studies of the school environment. The goal of this program for this type of environment is to help the faculty of the school redefine the purposes of the school, and to create feedback functions so that the organization can begin to assess the effects of their environment upon its members. For this type of social organization the period of preparation for the change program would be expected to be longer than the period of implementation. Because of the absence of organizational diversity, long periods of time would be expected to be required to interpret the program, to receive sanction from the faculty for the program, and to communicate the goals of the program. Following interpretation, the operation of the program can be expected to be implemented in a shorter period of time. In fact, the change agents for this program will be alert to insure that the services do not receive premature adoption, and the faculty absorbed and preoccupied with a newer ideology.

Evaluating the effects of interventions for the constant environment would assess the effects of the program upon the functions of the organization, particularly aspects of the school environment, such as use of resources, relationships to other community resources, how the organization plans for change, and how the school goes about developing mechanisms for increasing diversity.

CONCLUSIONS

The proposed interventions for these two types of schools are based upon a view of the social settings and the individual behavior of the members as interdependent. The interest in this work is in knowing as much about adaptive societies as adaptive persons. The approach to this integrative task is to study both processes in contrasting environments, and to learn how people emerge in changing societies, without limiting the development of either themselves or the evolution of the society.

W. Bennis cites A. N. Whitehead, who crisply sums it up:

The art of free society consists first in the maintenance of the symbolic code, and secondly in the fearlessness of revision ... Those societies which cannot combine reverence to their symbols with freedom of revision must ultimately decay (Bennis, 1966, p. 205) ...

BIBLIOGRAPHY

Ardrey, R. *The territorial imperative.* New York: Atheneum, 1966.
Barker, R. G. Ecology and motivation. In M. R. Jones (Ed.), *Nebraska Symposium on Motivation*, 1960. Lincoln: University of Nebraska Press, 1960. Pp. 1-49.
Barker, R. G., & Gump, P. V. *Big school, small school.* Stanford, Calif.: Stanford University Press, 1964.

Barker, R. G. Explorations in ecological psychology. *American Psychologist*, 1965, **20**, 1-14.

Becker, H. S., Blance, G., Hughes, E., & Strauss, A. *Boys in white: Student culture in medical school.* Chicago: The University of Chicago Press, 1961.

Bennis, W. G. *Changing organizations.* New York: McGraw-Hill, 1966.

Bredemeier, H. C. Proposal for an adequate socialization structure. In Group for the Advancement of Psychiatry (Ed.), *Urban America and the planning of mental health services.* Washington, D.C.: Group for the Advancement of Psychiatry, 1964. Pp. 447-469.

Brim, O. G., Jr., & Wheeler, S. *Socialization after childhood: Two essays.* New York: John Wiley, 1966.

Caplan, G. *Principles of preventive psychiatry.* New York: Basic Books, 1964.

Clarke, G. *Elements of ecology.* New York: John Wiley, 1954.

Dyckman, J. W. City planning and the treasury of science. In W. R. Ewald, Jr. (Ed.), *Environment for man: The next fifty years.* Bloomington, Ind.: Indiana University Press, 1967. Pp. 27-59.

Endler, N. S., & Hunt, J. McV. Sources of behavioral variance as measured by the S-R inventory of anxiousness. *Psychological Bulletin*, 1966, **65** (6), 336-346.

Geertz, C. *Agricultural involution: The process of ecological change in Indonesia.* Berkeley: University of California Press, 1963.

Katz, D., & Kahn, R. L. *The social psychology of organizations.* New York: John Wiley, 1966.

Kelly, J. G. Ecological constraints on mental health services. *American Psychologist*, 1966a, **21**, 535-539.

Kelly, J. G. Social adaptation to varied environments. Paper read at American Psychological Association meeting, New York, September, 1966b.

Kelly, J. G. Naturalistic observations and theory confirmation: An example. *Human Development*, 1967, **10**, 212-222.

Klein, D. C., & Lindemann, E. Preventive intervention in family crisis situations. In G. Caplan (Ed.), *Prevention of mental disorders in children.* New York: Basic Books, 1961. Pp. 283-306.

Lazarus, R. S. *Psychological stress and the coping process.* New York: McGraw-Hill, 1966.

Levins, R. The strategy of model building in population biology. *American Scientist*, 1966, **54**, 421-431.

Lewontin, R. C. The adaptations of populations to varying environments. *Cold Springs Harbor Symposium on Quantitative Biology*, 1958, **22**, 395-408.

Macfadyen, A. *Animal biology: Aims and methods.* London: Pitman, 1957.

Mechanic, D. *Students under stress: A study in the social psychology of adaptation.* New York: The Free Press, 1962.

Orth, C. D. *Social structure and learning climate: The first year at Harvard Business School.* Boston: Graduate School of Business Administration, Harvard University, 1963.

Pugh, D. S. Modern organization theory: A psychological and sociological study. *Psychological Bulletin*, 1966, **66**, 235-251.

Rotter, J. B. Generalized expectancies for internal versus external control of reinforcement. *Psychology Monographs*, 1966, **80** (1, All No. 609).

Simpson, G. G. Biology and the public good. *American Scientist*, 1967, **55**, 161-175.

Smith, R. L. *Ecology and field biology.* New York: Harper & Row, 1966.

Sommer, R. Small group ecology. *Psychological Bulletin,* 1967, **67,** 145-152.

Watt, K. E. F. (Ed.). *Systems analysis in ecology.* New York: Academic Press, 1966.

Williams, G. C. *Adaptation and natural selection: A critique of some current evolutionary thought.* Princeton, N.J.: Princeton University Press, 1966.

CHAPTER 9

Community Actions and the Prevention of Alcoholism

Nevitt Sanford

"Alcohol problems," "problem drinking," "alcoholism"—these are terms which, according to the Cooperative Commission on the Study of Alcoholism (Cooperative Commission, 1967), ought to be carefully distinguished. "Alcohol problems," the most inclusive conception, refers to all the issues and dilemmas that exist in connection with alcohol, not only to troublesome behavior accompanying or following the excessive use of alcohol but to such questions as:

—Why has American society been unable to arrive at any generally accepted standards or folkways concerning when, where, and how to drink?

—Why do the institutions and agencies that seek to cope with alcohol problems so often find themselves in conflict?

—Why does the socially damaging behavior that sometimes follows the use of alcohol receive less attention than it should from responsible lay and professional people?

"Problem drinking" is "a repetitive use of beverage alcohol causing physical, psychological, or social harm to the drinker or to others" (Cooperative Commission, 1967, p. 37), while "alcoholism" is a type of problem drinking "in which an individual has lost control over his alcohol intake in the sense that he is consistently unable to refrain from drinking or to stop drinking before getting intoxicated" (Cooperative Commission, 1967, p. 39).

This chapter will focus on the prevention of alcoholism. We must recognize, however, that alcohol problems are interrelated and that each of them exists within a context of other problems. Consequently, most measures for the prevention of alcoholism are nonspecific, in the sense that they can be expected to affect other problems as well. At the same time, there are various actions that could help prevent other alcohol problems—for example, "driving under the influence"—but which would have little to do with the prevention of alcoholism. Hence, the discussion here may be kept within reasonable limits by restricting it to this one type of problem drinking.

Actions to prevent alcoholism should be guided by knowledge of its causes but, unfortunately, such knowledge leaves much to be desired. That the condition (or conditions) is due to a combination of biological, psychological, and social causes is generally agreed upon; yet it still happens that cases are sorted out according to the factor, in one or another of these areas, that is believed to be the key. In one case, a genetically determined metabolic deficiency is said to be the cause; in another, a personality problem generated in early childhood; and in still another, a social group's assigning the label "drunkard" to a steady drinker and then rewarding him for taking this role. The practice is favored by the fact that for any case of persistent problem drinking a resourceful specialist in biology, or psychology, or sociology can produce a plausible explanation in terms of his discipline. An opinion that has gained wide acceptance among experts is that no one single factor by itself will bring about alcoholism, although it is to be admitted that in different cases different kinds of factors will be more important than others. Even if it should be demonstrated that some people come into the world with some kind of metabolic deficit that renders them especially susceptible to certain bodily effects when they consume alcohol, we should not regard this as a sole cause of later alcoholism. Genetic and environmental factors begin their interactions early, even in utero, and it is highly unlikely that any identifiable bodily or behavioral process in an adolescent or adult can be ascribed solely to factors of one or the other sort. A person might have such a deficiency and, in addition, a deep-seated emotional problem generated in early childhood, but this would not necessarily make him an addicted drinker either, for he might develop various other symptoms instead of alcoholism. If such a person encountered crises in his later life, the chances of his becoming alcoholic would be increased, but certainly not guaranteed. Probably, in addition, such a person would have to grow up in a culture in which there were pressures both to drink and not to drink, and an absence of agreed norms for ways of drinking. It seems probable that in any case of alcoholism all of these kinds of factors have been present in complicated interrelationships.

This view of the matter presents a formidable challenge to anyone interested in prevention. The outlook would be discouraging indeed if action had to await precise knowledge of causation. But, as public-health work has shown, effective action against a disease or disorder may be taken even though we do not know just how that condition is caused. If it is assumed, as we have just done in the case of alcoholism, that a disease or disorder is caused by a chain of events involving a number of factors, then it follows that radical modification in one of the factors or even slight modification in some of them can reduce the rate at which that disease or disorder appears in a population.

On the basis of the above formulation concerning the causes of alcoholism, three kinds of preventive actions can be distinguished: (1) reducing bodily susceptibilities, (2) improving mental health, and (3) altering drinking patterns.

Concerning (1), little can be said, for virtually nothing is known about specific metabolic or nutritional deficiencies that could lead to a person's becoming alcoholic. About the only primary preventive measure that can be proposed at this time is the completely nonspecific one of insuring that everybody has an adequate diet. At the same time, however, there is no doubt that people differ in their physiological reactions to alcohol, and we may well believe that specific metabolic or nutritional factors in alcoholism will eventually be discovered. There are psychologically healthy people who know that alcohol has a special physiological significance for them. They know that, where drugs are concerned, one man's meat is another man's poison, and that for them alcohol is "it." They say they would surely take to it in a big way should personal problems become severe—the price of individual psychotherapy being what it is. Perhaps it would be good if these people could be made to resemble more closely those other mentally healthy people who believe—let's assume with good reason—that their physiology protects them from becoming problem drinkers: they become ill or drowsy or have unpleasant sensations before they consume enough alcohol to do them any "good"—or any harm.

The study of abstainers and of people with low tolerance for alcohol might quite conceivably teach us something about how the ways in which individuals absorb or metabolize alcohol might be altered to their advantage—assuming, of course, that they are provided with some means other than drinking for dealing with severe psychological stress.

PREVENTION THROUGH IMPROVING MENTAL HEALTH

It is a safe assumption that, in a great many cases of alcoholism, personal problems and tensions or disturbed functioning of the personality are among the major determining factors, and that these factors are at work as contributing or precipitating factors in virtually all cases found in our society. It follows from this that rates of alcohol problems would be reduced if means could be found for bringing about a general improvement in the mental health of our population.

Personality malfunction of the sort that could help induce problem drinking is usually due in some part to the impact of experiences in childhood and in some part to critical situations in the individual's life after he is old enough to start drinking. We must be concerned in the first place, then, with preventing disturbances in childhood (for example, through actions to improve family relations or to equip mothers to deal with crises in the life of the child) and with providing the kind of child training and education that can develop personalities capable of coping with emotional crises as they arise. We should not, however, put all the emphasis on childhood. We should assume that the personality-forming years extend through adolescence and into young adulthood, that it is possible during these periods to prepare people for dealing with anticipated crises and to introduce educational measures that can further develop the adaptive capacities of the individual.

Fostering mental health is also a matter of improving the conditions of life—whatever the age of the individual—so that too many severe crises do not occur and so that, when they do, the environment offers support and means for coping with the crises. Particular attention has to be given to people who live in potentially unhealthy or dangerous situations, for example, unattached men living in isolation or men who have recently retired from the army (with consequent loss of security, status, and sense of usefulness).

It seems obvious that if actions of these general kinds reduced rates of alcoholism, they would be likely to reduce rates of other illnesses and disorders as well; and that actions which were effective in respect to other illnesses and disorders would very probably reduce rates of problem drinking.

This conclusion is in keeping with the fact that no "alcoholic personality" has been found. This is not to say that there is no evidence that certain deep-seated personality dispositions (for example, oral fixation, emotional dependence, inadequate self-esteem, or manic-depressive tendencies) dispose to alcoholism; it is rather that all known dispositions of this kind might express themselves in other ways as well.

What can be said, then, about preventing alcoholism through fostering mental health does not differ essentially from what can be said about preventing delinquency or neurosis or other kinds of mental disorders. Alcohol specialists have to make common cause with all specialists who work toward the improvement of mental health; and since this is the major concern of other chapters in this book, it need not be discussed here.

There is, however, one type of case in which efforts to improve the psychological functioning of people may be directed specifically to alcoholism. This is the case in which the individual has begun to show early signs of later trouble with alcohol or appears to be in the early stages of alcoholism. Intervention with a view to preventing the condition from developing further would be an example of *secondary prevention*—to use another term borrowed from the field of public health. Secondary prevention cannot be sharply separated from treatment and rehabilitation, for if the object of intervention is to prevent a diagnosed condition from developing into something worse then, logically, all treatment is preventive. Suppose, however, it should be found in a population that a relatively large number of people exhibited, in their behavior or in their situation, problematic conditions that were known to be, in general, predisposing to alcoholism and were already causing some trouble. And suppose that the measures chosen to remedy these conditions were directed to all these people as a group and involved changing features of an environment that they all shared. It would seem inappropriate to call these measures "treatment."

An example of specific secondary prevention would be a program of testing for early signs of trouble with alcohol instituted at a school or college, the whole student population being given physiological tests. It might be revealed that 15 per cent (or several hundred students) showed characteristics known to be associated with the later development of alcoholism. A program of interviewing that consisted mainly in informing these students of their physiological liabilities and in opening the way to future counseling (should they desire it) would, it seems, be best conceived as secondary prevention. The students, we are assuming, would not, in the first instance at least, have asked for treatment, nor would the interviewing be permitted to develop into a psychotherapeutic relationship.

If a testing program should be made the basis for an effort to inform the whole school or college community about alcohol or to develop more mature attitudes around drinking, we would have an instance of primary prevention. But we would expect those who already had problems to receive the most benefit from it; for them, in other words, the preventive activity directed to populations that include people who already have mild symptoms is one of the best forms of secondary prevention. The distinction between primary and secondary prevention here becomes blurred, although it is clear that we are not talking about treatment.

PREVENTION THROUGH ALTERING DRINKING PATTERNS

We have said that even though a person has a bodily constitution and a personality structure that favors addiction to alcohol, his actually becoming alcoholic would still depend heavily upon factors in his environment. What do we have in mind? For one thing, we are thinking of attitudes, beliefs, and practices concerning alcohol that are embedded in our culture and that tend to bring alcohol to the forefront of the individual's attention and to favor its use as a means for altering various kinds of unpleasant psychological states. Again, there are in our culture prevalent beliefs about and attitudes toward alcohol that tend to give it special significance for individuals with particular kinds of psychological problems. For example, heavy drinking is widely regarded, in our culture, as a sign of "manliness." We should expect, therefore, that adolescents and young men who have worries about their manhood would naturally tend to choose this easy and culturally prescribed way of asserting their masculinity. To take another example, we have seen that in our culture drinking often tends to be invested with the same kind of guilt and fascination as does sex. If an individual, before he has learned to control his sexuality, is taught to believe that all sexual behavior is wrong, we do not expect him to give up sexuality altogether. Rather, we expect him to feel guilty about it, at best to delay heterosexual activity until a suitable time, at most to develop pathological sexual attitudes and practices. Similarly with drinking. If young people are taught that alcohol is a product of the devil and that they should feel guilty for so much as thinking of it, we might produce some total abstainers among them; but in a country in which perhaps 75 per cent of the adult population drink, a more likely outcome is what we in fact have: a large number of pathological drinkers.

We consider, too, the probability that some people become steady and heavy drinkers without predisposing constitutional or personality factors, but just because they participate in a culture or subculture in which heavy drinking is expected of everyone. If a person who has acquired this pattern in these circumstances should fall upon evil days, be faced with an emotional crisis or with mounting strains—and if his drinking did not have any meaningful place in his personality organization or self-conception—resort to drinking-for-relief would not be surprising.

Action or policy with respect to drinking must be based on knowledge of the consequences of particular patterns of drinking or abstaining, whether or not they favor the attainment of long-range social or individual goals. What is needed, both for further research and as a guide to action, is a typology of drinking and abstaining that is based on the relations of the practice to the group's or to the individual's purposes, functioning, and development. The following scheme of "ideal types" of drinking behavior owes more to field observations and individual case studies than to research employing formal designs. It differs from drinking typologies presented in the literature in two ways: first, for reasons just given, the present tentative scheme is frankly normative, while almost all other typologies have aimed at value-free description; and, second, the same general theoretical framework is used in formulating both group and individual practices. Both groups and individuals are systems and both may be viewed in a developmental perspective. The scheme owes most to Fallding (1964);

indeed, his scheme could be used for our present purposes if it were less complex and if it lent itself to the analysis of individual functioning.

Group Practices

By attending to the relations of a drinking practice to a group's purposes, functioning, and development, we may distinguish three types of drinking: escapist, facilitative, and integrative.

Escapist drinking in a social group would be a shared way of trying to get away from shared unpleasant or frustrating states or situations. Examples would be drinking to relieve boredom or emptiness; to retreat from too much authority or restriction; to overcome anxiety, inadequacy, or inferiority; to alleviate other kinds of harsh reality, for example, the sense of being "trapped" in a system of work or social relations. Drinking to keep up with the fashion, to meet conformity pressures, or to maintain status belong in this category if we consider that group members want to escape feeling alone or outcast or experiencing a lowered status.

Facilitative drinking can break down coldness or reserve in a social group and help induce conviviality. It increases the intensity of communication, favors the free flow of information, and thus helps people to get acquainted. There is some evidence that in complicated social structures, such as a business organization or a hospital, it can be an aid to communication among people of different statuses and thus make the system function more smoothly.

Integrative drinking is drinking which has a meaningful place within a larger organization of processes; it contributes something to that organization and to the achievement of some of its purposes, but it is not essential to the existence of that organization. The sensory pleasure in drinking would be enhanced by its embeddedness in the social setting, but the main experience of pleasure would proceed from the total situation of which drinking was a part. For example, it might, as in ceremonial drinking, symbolize pre-existing community and thus contribute to the forging of greater solidarity. But it would not be relied upon to create community where none existed before. To be integrative, drinking need not have any explicitly social purpose; it would only have to have a meaningful place—an appropriate but not necessary place—within a set of activities that is consistent with social and individual well-being. It is not necessarily moderate in amount. Drinking to intoxication, or near intoxication, or with a view to becoming intoxicated would qualify, provided the time, place, and setting were appropriate.

Abstaining, like drinking, should be looked at with attention to its context and meaning. There are cases in which abstaining is an integral part of culturewide beliefs and ways, which it favors and by which it is sustained. The Hopi Indians, for example, in maintaining prohibition throughout their society for many years, were deliberately expressing their rejection of the white man's ways and forging solidarity within the community.

Abstinence in a social group begins to take on the aspect of escapism when the belief system of that group is threatened by all kinds of contrary beliefs in its surround, so that it becomes necessary for the group to insist rigidly upon adherence to the letter of all of its laws and to express hostility toward all surrounding groups whose ways are different.

Individual Patterns

The very numerous forms of individual drinking, depending on how drinking relates to the whole personality and its manifold needs, may be called escapist, facilitative, or integrative. These terms have essentially the same meanings here as in the discussion of group practices, only now the individual personality is the "system" with whose purposes, functions, and development we are concerned.

Escapist drinking, as the term implies, is drinking to avoid the pains of frustration, anxiety, or emotional stress, and drinking to gain by a short-cut the gratification of impulses that cannot be admitted into the conscious ego. The problems that cause pain are real, and the relief found in drinking is genuine; the trouble is that the relief can be only temporary, and the drinking contributes nothing to the solution of the problems. Indeed, it usually stands in the way of what might be effective means for coping.

A drinking pattern can be classified as escapist on the basis of its relations to personality processes before there is any question of a medical diagnosis of alcoholism and without attention to the future course of the drinking. For example, if we know that a fraternity boy drinks heavily in order to overcome doubts about his masculinity, we call that drinking escapist even though its manifest pattern does not differ from the norm for his house, and even though we have reason to believe the pattern will change as he gains greater security in his male identity. With individuals, as with social groups, the use of alcohol as a means for escaping temporary tensions may not be the least adaptive stratagem that could be found, nor does their use of this stratagem necessarily set in motion irreversible processes.

In the case just cited, the drinking is to escape the anxiety occasioned by an unconscious conflict. We also class as escapist those forms of drinking that express needs or fantasies that are barred from consciousness. Since in our culture drinking often symbolizes something "bad" (either because the individual has connected it with repressed impulses or because he has been brought up to believe it is bad in and of itself), a common defense is deliberately to isolate the drinking from the self or otherwise to render it meaningless—as when, in American movies, drinking is made to appear as casual as lighting a cigarette and is not supposed to have any effects one way or the other.

Facilitative drinking is widely acclaimed in our society as a means for overcoming shyness, acquiring courage to face a difficult situation, achieving a change of mood, relaxing after a period of stress, and producing various other desired states or effects in the individual. Often, facilitative drinking is actually the rationalization of escapist drinking, but it does appear that there are situations in which drinking may be genuinely facilitative in the sense that it serves nondestructive purposes of the individual and does not work against the integration of the personality. If there is evidence that the activities and outcomes facilitated are increasingly capable of realization without drinking, while they *and* the drinking become more pleasurable in association, then there is movement toward integration. If, on the other hand, no signs of such change are observed, it may be that the real source of the shyness is being further obscured and cut off from the rest of the personality and, hence, that there is movement toward disintegrative or escapist drinking.

Integrative drinking has a meaningful place within a larger process, by which it is rendered more satisfying and which it enhances. It is not a necessity; it does not interfere seriously with the satisfaction of other needs; it has a place in the conscious self; it is not engaged in automatically or against the will; and it is not followed by regret.

The essential object of integrative drinking is pleasure. As with the indulgence of the senses generally, the deepest and most durable satisfaction from drinking comes when it is integrated with the expression of other needs, as in friendship and conviviality, or as in connoisseurship, where a whole complex of sensations and cognitions is evoked. Where drinking is integrated with other needs in the conscious ego, the individual may, so to speak, throw himself into the act and thus find deep satisfaction just because a variety of needs are being expressed together. Ego development is here of crucial importance. The individual could not tie in his drinking with other needs unless these needs had been developed and had found a place in the conscious ego, nor could the ego abandon itself to pleasure in the way being suggested here unless it possessed enough flexibility to give assurance that it could return to its usual state.

Abstaining in the individual could be regarded as integrative when that individual belonged to an abstaining culture or subculture and had decided, after deliberation, that he preferred to maintain this particular tenet of the belief system out of loyalty to the group and out of the feeling that abstaining was integral to the belief system that he wished to support. Abstaining might be facilitative of some particular purpose of the individual, as in an athlete who had become convinced that drinking would prevent him from doing his best.

Abstaining begins to take on the features of escapism when it expresses for the individual one side of a deep-seated conflict. He might unconsciously wish to drink because drinking symbolizes for him impulses that are ordinarily forbidden expression and must be restrained at all costs. In these circumstances the individual must struggle to avoid even the thought of drinking, and he may help his cause by trying to see to it that no one else drinks either.

It is clear then that we cannot take up a position with respect to abstaining per se, either on the part of a group or on the part of an individual. With abstinence, as with drinking, our basic concern is with the promotion of integration both in the social group and in the individual personality.

We come then to the conclusion that community action to prevent alcoholism must be directed, first of all, to cultural change. And if we ask about the direction of cultural change, the answer must be: toward patterns that favor individual development. Assuming that ours will continue to be predominantly a "drinking" culture, we want an alcohol policy that will favor the integratedness of group drinking practices. We may further assume that integratedness in society's drinking practices will help its youthful members to integrate their drinking with their personalities. This outcome would not be inevitable, however; for just as some mentally healthy individuals could be led into difficulties in a society in which pathological drinking patterns prevailed, so some individuals would find in alcohol a means for escaping personal problems even though their society's drinking patterns are highly integrative. We must, therefore, in addition to promoting integratedness in group drinking practices, plan actions specifically directed to the integration of drinking in the individual personality.

Actions toward these ends may be classed under three general headings: (1) enlightenment in society, (2) the regulation of trade, and (3) alcohol education in the schools. These kinds of actions are interrelated and interacting, as we shall see.

PREVENTION THROUGH ENLIGHTENMENT IN SOCIETY

There is need for actions that can help add awareness, meaningfulness, and understanding on the part of the general public to the whole phenomenon of drinking. It follows from what has been said about types of drinking that we cannot advocate, for those who drink, a particular mode of drinking or the use of a particular beverage, because everything depends upon the meaning of drinking and the context in which it occurs. We can, however, urge that integration be promoted and escapism discouraged, and that the particular norms generated be in keeping with this general orientation.

Public discussion can help to overcome the "conspiracy of silence" about drinking. It must be shown that everything about alcohol and drinking can be discussed, and that all the issues arising in connection with this subject have to be settled. There are myths to be exposed, and inappropriate or unworthy practices to be criticized. In general, there must be discussion directed to showing how attitudes and behavior with respect to alcohol can be brought into line with the dominant values of our culture—values that include maximum freedom of choice for the individual.

To further public discussion, there is need for a literature that is free of sanctimoniousness, that focuses on drinking rather than on alcoholism, and that appeals to the educated reader—the likely molder of opinion. This literature would tie in drinking and alcohol-related problems with the existing interests of people who read and who take some responsibility for what happens in our society. The intellectual challenges of alcohol problems would be accented. The appeal to community leaders might well be less on the basis that alcohol problems are serious and costly (there are many such problems) and more on the basis that they are interesting and intellectually challenging.

The existence of suitable literature would not, of course, suffice to create the kind of interest and excitement necessary to assure its being read—to say nothing of setting social change in motion. There would still be a need to create issues that directly affect the public. For example, the organized alcohol educators, or some college authorities—fed up at last with the hypocrisy in which they participate—might start agitating for repeal of the legal-age limitation. Whether or not they got anywhere with the state legislatures, they could take advantage of the excitement generated to gain attention for their messages concerning acceptable and unacceptable drinking, the problems of youth in our society, and so on.

When the kind of enlightenment and atmosphere of freedom here being urged had been attained, the temperance point of view would receive the same hearing as others, and individuals who did not wish to drink would be free of social pressure to do so. Also, the task of alcohol education in the schools would be very different from what it is now. It would be largely a matter of informal socialization; the necessary facts about the effects of alcohol and the etiology of problem drinking would be acquired quickly and easily; and conflicts about drinking would be utilized in the interests of education for individual development.

PREVENTION THROUGH REGULATION OF TRADE

The Cooperative Commission on the Study of Alcoholism has suggested a number of ways in which changes in laws and policies might reduce escapist and promote integrative drinking (Cooperative Commission, 1967, pp. 138-152). And Wilkinson (in press), a member of the commission's staff, has discussed these suggestions, and others of his own, in detail. Wilkinson has summarized these suggestions as follows:

—Removal of many restrictions, especially in retailing and advertising, that stigmatize alcohol (and pester the trade).

—Tax changes and promotion that help shift consumption to lighter proof drinks, associated with meals and snacks; licensing policies and promotion that associate alcohol definitely with meals in the home and in restaurants.

—Licensing laws and other measures that move alcohol away from an emphasis on drinking-only into settings and activities enjoyed by the whole family together: sports events, resorts (carefully scrutinized), bowling alleys, theaters, and so on.

—Requirements and inducements that change taverns from dark and furtive haunts to well-lit, cheerful places where people can get food as well as drink.

—Commercial advertising policies, encouraged by government regulation, which portray alcohol not as a lyrical or he-man symbol but as a part of moderate, if attractive, everyday living, taken with family and friends in circumstances of restraint. Women and children portrayed in or near drinking scenes, in such a way that they suggest restraint (Wilkinson, in press).

In connection with this last suggestion, it is interesting to note that liquor advertisements do not depict women in the act of drinking (a rule of the Alcohol and Tobacco Tax Division). This is a nice expression of the idea, found almost universally in history and in preliterate cultures of the present day, that drinking belongs essentially to the sphere of the male. The ATTD is here participating in a strong trend in our culture and at the same time encouraging the liquor industry to exploit that trend. There is good reason to believe that more alcohol per individual is consumed, other things being equal, in all-male settings and in settings where men take the lead than in mixed groups. It also seems highly likely that this advertising, besides helping to perpetuate an authoritarian or feudalistic trend in our culture, favors problem drinking. Such advertising encourages drinking to display virility on the part of men, and it promotes the idea that drinking on the part of women is still somewhat daring or adventurous, something that "ladies" do not do. What does the industry gain, or expect to gain, by adhering to these anachronistic notions and images? Perhaps it has shrewdly calculated that this approach sells more alcohol to men, while actually doing nothing to restrict consumption on the part of women. Or perhaps here, as elsewhere, it simply pays its respects to what are supposed to be the prevailing norms.

The Cooperative Commission, with a view particularly to helping young people "to adapt themselves to a predominantly 'drinking society' "—in our terms, to integrate drinking into the personality—has also suggested that all age restrictions for alcohol "probably should be eliminated" and that for the time being a minimum age of 18 for public drinking or purchase (it is presently 21 in most states) might be adopted. The chief arguments are that since more than 75 per cent of high-school students report that they have had alcoholic beverages more than once, the age limit of 21 is largely unenforceable and creates a hypocritical situation, and that the lower limit—or none at all—would give youth an opportunity to learn to drink integratively while reducing the frequency with which they begin drinking furtively or in ways that signify rebellion or the partaking of "forbidden fruit."

This suggestion of the Cooperative Commission may be further supported on the basis of the theory of personality development —the same theory that underlies the suggestions offered in the following section, on alcohol education in schools.

PREVENTION THROUGH ALCOHOL EDUCATION IN SCHOOLS

According to theory, highly developed individuals are able to integrate actions and experiences with their egos.

Whether or not a particular action or experience will be so integrated depends both on the degree of the ego's development (how extensive and complex it is) and on the nature of the action or experience, that is, on how understandable, how consistent with pre-existing structures, or how unanticipated or shocking it is. A child, whose ego is not yet well developed, would have no trouble integrating with his ego the experience of sipping wine with his family, who were drinking integratively. But if he witnessed drunkenness and riotous behavior on the part of his family or was seduced into drinking by older children in an atmosphere of surreptitious rebellion, he would be very likely to associate drinking with tendencies that children ordinarily exclude from the ego. A teenager who had been taught from childhood that drinking was a sin would need a more fully developed personality structure in order to integrate it with his own drinking experiences than would a teenager who believed that drinking was a normal adult activity. A college freshman who had grown up in an abstaining family and community, and who more or less automatically adopted abstinence as a way of life, would have more trouble resisting pressures to drink than would a freshman who knew the facts about alcohol and drinking and had given the matter serious thought—who, in other words, was well started in the direction of integrating his abstaining behavior with his developing ego.

Since alcohol, when taken in more than very moderate amounts, has the capacity to release impulses, drinking will raise for most teenagers who experiment with it the general issue of impulse control. Efforts are often made by groups who would influence drinking practices in our society to remove drinking from the context of impulse expression by urging that it be "moderate," "reasonable," "responsible," and so on. What this approach often means is that, even though one drinks, the characteristic effects of alcohol are to be avoided. This is accomplished by the child who sips wine with his parents, the man who takes sufficient food with his beer, the lady who takes a cocktail at a party but has learned to stop drinking before its effects are experienced. There is a place for these kinds of "dry" drinking, this use of alcohol as a beverage like any other. If, however, the drinking is an expression of a general "antipleasure ideology," it cannot qualify as integrative drinking. The point is that most people who enjoy drinking want sometimes to be immoderate and, temporarily, free of the requirements of reason and responsibility. Within limits, it is probably a good thing to show young people that beverage alcohol is perfectly natural, nothing to get excited about, something (as the liquor ads say) that good consumers buy and consume as they do everything else that is advertised. But since drinking for pleasure is essentially a matter of impulse expression, and will be experienced as such by teenagers who drink, it would seem the better part of wisdom to help young people, through education, to integrate their impulses with their ego, so that they may enjoy life, avoiding both overrigid restrictions on themselves and damaging outbreaks of what they have been forbidden.

Alcohol education, then, has the dual goal of preparing young people for the experiences that are to come and of assuring that what they experience is assimilable. The former may be promoted through such procedures as presenting some facts about the effects of alcohol before drinking begins or offering some anticipatory counseling. The latter could be accomplished by avoiding the definition of alcohol as something fearful and of drinking as sinful, and by encouraging young people who are going to drink to delay the beginning of impulse-expressive drinking until there is a likelihood that their experiences will be pleasant and not regrettable.

To achieve this dual goal, alcohol education must be guided by a conception of stages of personality development. Children of elementary-school age might well be given some basic facts about alcohol and drinking; and there should certainly be arrangements for answering all their questions about these subjects. This introduction would help to prepare them for their teenage experiences; but we should not expect these facts to be very meaningful to them or this knowledge to be a large factor in determining their later behavior.

In the case of teenagers, the major implication of the theory offered here is that they should be encouraged and helped to wait before beginning the kind of drinking that is impulse-releasing— insofar as waiting is possible. Those parents who feel "in their bones" that age 14 is too young for drinking in groups away from home have the right instinct. We cannot expect drinking, that is expressive of impulses, to be integrated in the personality until the personality has become relatively well developed. Rather we expect, and too often find, that when impulse-expressive drinking is begun too early, it is likely to become isolated from the personality and to take on meanings that make its later integration difficult or impossible. When this happens, the individual reduces his chances of finding genuine pleasure in drinking later on. Moreover, the development of the personality may be impaired. It must be admitted that not all who in the past advocated a 21-year-old limitation were either prohibitionist or seriously misguided. The effort to define drinking as an adult activity still has much to recommend it. It is a sound general principle that the meaningfulness and satisfaction of life's experiences are, within limits, greater when the context to which they are to be assimilated is broader and richer. The question is, When does adulthood begin? And how do we, a society that has smudged over all boundaries separating youth and age, prevent children from acting as if they were grown-up, thereby missing the joys of their innocence and spoiling their chances of great experiences later on? We can at least accent the idea of *readiness*, and say with assurance that an 18-year-old is more ready than a 14-year-old. This accent on readiness would help parents, educators, and teenagers to make a case for waiting, without being moralistic and without arousing the fears associated with ideas about damage to physical health.

It is not to be expected that teenagers or college students will immediately embrace the ethics of integration. These young people focus on what adults do, rather than on what they say, and the idea of postponement, even when it is in the interest of greater satisfaction later on, is likely to be regarded as another, perhaps more subtle proscription. Happily, these young people are not the final arbiters in such matters. Studies have shown that a majority of them, if a vote were taken, would favor not only the 21-year-old limitation on the purchase of alcoholic beverages but also other rules as strict as those now on the books. Our youth are not, by and large, unhappy about the present situation; as college students are fond of saying, "The administration has the rules and we have the booze." Young people do not automatically blossom forth with personal responsibility and consistent value orientations as soon as they are given the freedom to do so. These virtues, like most others, have to be cultivated through education; and education has to be guided by conceptions of what young people need for their development rather than by what they say they want at particular times. Often, they want to be very moral, and they look to the adult community for standards. On such occasions, it would appear far better to offer them, as the ideal, the morality of personality integration than to uphold authoritarian systems, which young people naturally favor as a ready means for controlling their impulses.

What has just been said is an example of the characteristic lack of personality integration found in normal adolescents. This is no indication of the level of integration to be attained later on. Development entails differentiation as well as integration, and there is always a certain tension between the two processes. To become complex personalities, adolescents must try a wide range of styles, identities, roles, and other behavior patterns—some of which are inconsistent, seem foreign to them, and are otherwise startling to their parents and other adults. We cannot expect these various facets to be integrated now; but we can see to it that the capacity for later integration, which is a matter of ego development, is nurtured through education.

The sections below discuss activities that might well be undertaken by alcohol educators, but, hopefully, they will be undertaken by other educators as well. The activities are directed to the more specific aims of alcohol education, but they should be of general benefit to individual students at the high-school as well as college level.

Activities of the School as a Whole

The school is best conceived as a whole, with all of its activities (not just those of the classroom) viewed as educational and evaluated in terms of what they contribute, or fail to contribute, to individual development. There are different kinds of schools, each with a social structure, a pattern of roles and functions designed, in the first instance, to carry out educational policies; and each with a culture, a "climate" of belief and value orientation, in whose context prevailing attitudes and practices with respect to drinking are to be understood.

Attitudes, standards, and practices with respect to drinking are so largely a reflection of a more general value orientation within a school that knowing the former, one could predict the latter with some accuracy. If, for example, a school persisted in teaching only the dangers of alcohol while ignoring the fact that a substantial minority of the students were drinking surreptitiously, one could be reasonably certain that it was participating in a general ideology, in accordance with which a wide range of puritanical or authoritarian standards was officially upheld while behavior contrary to the standards was more or less tolerated so long as it did not break into the open. The drinking behavior of the students in such a school, and the task of alcohol education, would be radically different from what would be the case in a school in an upper-middle-class district of a city where most of the parents had college degrees and prided themselves on their enlightenment. The difference would be like that between a large metropolitan university and a small private college to which parents sent their sons and daughters in the hope that the small school would provide a protected environment.

The drinking behavior of the students in a particular school, together with the problem of its modification, depends not only on the surrounding adult culture, but on the student culture or, possibly, subcultures of that school. Adolescents develop their own ways of dealing with our cultural confusion about alcohol and with the other pressures of their situation; and some of these ways, aided by the conformity needs of adolescents, may become dominating in a given institution. For example, fairly hard-drinking social clubs might set the general tone.

Who sets the tone in a given school depends on the structure of student society: the number of social clubs, their status, the proportion of students who belong to these organizations, the number and strength of competing student organizations, and so on. This structure depends in turn on such factors as the composition of the student body and the policies of the school administration respecting student organizations.

The content of the student drinking culture depends not only on what parents and school officials do and say about drinking, but on structural features of the particular school program. Some schools, through the rigor of their academic programs and the rigidity of their bureaucracies, generate a great deal of tension in their students. Drinking, by individuals and groups, has become a not uncommon way of relieving tension. Its frequency and intensity will depend on the availability of other ways of "letting off steam" or satisfying the needs served by inappropriate drinking, and on the accessibility of adults with whom the young people involved might talk about their problems.

The school administration must understand the social context of student drinking and the institutional structure in which alcohol education must take place; and it must use this understanding both in its "handling" of crises and in its planning of actions to improve the whole system.

No amount of sound instruction in classrooms could undo the harm caused by an administration that displayed for students a wide gap between official position and actual practice, and thus confirmed their worst suspicions of adult hypocrisy. Equally destructive is the administration that, through its reaction to some breach of the rules, showed that it was unable to face alcohol issues or was willing to sacrifice the integrity of individual students in the interest of the school's "image." For that matter, it is hard to see how there could be sound instruction in the classroom unless the administration were willing to support teachers who got into trouble with parents or school boards because of their boldness in discussing controversial questions. On the other hand, the school administration is in an excellent position to show young people how emotion-laden issues can be faced in an intelligent and constructive way.

It is up to the school administration to create a context in which alcohol education, as it has been conceived here, might go forward. Most important is genuine communication with students, which is not only a first essential of alcohol education, but a basic requirement for general education. By listening to students, the educator learns what their needs are and develops ideas about what educational procedures are likely to be effective. He also creates in students receptivity to what he has to say. By being honest with students—and in the area of alcohol issues, honesty may include revealing something of what *his* dilemmas are—the educator provides a valuable lesson in morality. Alcohol issues and rules about drinking are particularly good topics for open discussion just because they are controversial and so frequently the prey of double-talk. Such discussion can teach much about the complexity of social processes, the necessity of rules, the differing responsibilities of adults and youth, and the intelligent approach to ethical issues.

The Teacher's Role and Preparation

Just as alcohol education is part of good general education, so the teacher who is good at dealing with alcohol and drinking is first of all a good teacher. Alcohol education in schools will improve as teacher training improves.

The teacher with responsibility for alcohol and drinking education must know how to deal with controversial subjects and how to induce students to talk about matters that concern them. He must be interested in students as individuals, not afraid of (or easily annoyed by) the noisy or deviant ones, and have some general knowledge of personality development. But these are essentials of all good teaching. This kind of skill, knowledge, and interest may be of greater importance in "education for living" than in traditional academic fields, but it is found in some teachers in all fields, and it will most certainly serve all teachers well.

The preparation of teachers, therefore, should include experience in college or university classrooms where controversial subjects were effectively treated. Prospective teachers should also have the experience of leading discussions of such subjects in their own practice teaching. All teachers should be familiar with the basic facts and principles of personality development, so that they understand how intellectual capacities develop in pace with the rest of the personality. All should be sensitive to interpersonal relations in the classroom, to their own feelings, and to those of their students. Larger infusions of developmental and social psychology and of sociology into teacher-training programs, in addition to improved general education, would help teachers acquire the right orientation to students and learning.

All teachers should know the basic facts about alcohol, drinking, and alcoholism; at the least, they should know what we are here proposing that all high-school students learn. Any teacher, and particularly the teacher in whom students have confidence, may be called upon at any time to discuss alcohol-related problems with students. And imaginative teachers in many fields can make their courses more interesting and touch the concerns of the students by using alcohol-related phenomena to illustrate biological, psychological, sociological, or philosophical principles they seek to put across.

Alcohol-related phenomena fit better naturally into some areas of the college and teacher-training curricula than into others. Teachers who are preparing for careers in such fields as health education, social studies, or contemporary problems may be expected to be more "expert" in alcohol matters than their colleagues in other fields. These teachers might well become the authorities on the subject at their schools, keeping up with the research in the field and being prepared to offer information to their fellow teachers. The task of gaining for alcohol problems a larger place in the specialized areas just mentioned is essentially the same as that of gaining for this subject a proper place in school and college curricula generally. It is a matter of overcoming our culturewide resistance to talking about the subject, arousing interest in it and showing its connectedness with various fields of inquiry.

School administrations, school boards, and state officials who have become aware of the importance of alcohol problems will not want to wait until a new generation of teachers has been trained; they will wish, instead, to help those now teaching to do a better job with the subject.

School authorities should in no case leave the matter in the hands of teachers who have a special interest in the subject because of their "dry" background, first-hand acquaintance with the destructiveness of alcoholism, or affiliation with organizations promoting a particular point of view. Such teachers have every right to be heard, and they may render service by goading the authorities into action; moreover, students should be exposed to the point of view of such teachers. But if this is the only point of view students hear expressed, they are not being educated about alcohol.

Probably the best course would be to persuade more teachers who understand young people and enjoy free discussion of controversial issues to include alcohol problems among the subjects they take up with students. These teachers can easily brush up their knowledge of the subject, for the basic information about drinking behavior, the effects of alcohol, and alcoholism does not constitute a large body of knowledge—particularly that portion relevant to the concerns of young people and suitable for presentation in high-school classrooms.

To know the basic facts about alcohol and alcohol-related problems is one thing; to understand the workings of a society such as ours and how students develop within it (the context within which alcohol-related problems must be viewed) is something else. Here are areas of inquiry that teachers bent on improving their work as educators will find inexhaustible.

There are many arrangements by which practicing teachers may receive further training: summer schools, summer institutes and workshops, weekend seminars, visits to the school—for lectures, seminars, and discussions—by scientists and professional people, and so on. It is no longer difficult to make such arrangements with a focus on alcohol problems, but it should be emphasized that learning the facts about such problems is of small significance compared with learning how to be a good teacher.

The problem is to persuade teachers to take advantage of those arrangements. It is like the problem of inducing students to attend a lecture on alcoholism. If attendance is optional, only those already converted will attend; if it is compulsory, nobody will listen. Here the administration must be aware of its responsibility for creating a context for alcohol education and it will do well to act with knowledge of the social structure of the particular school. Teachers who have traditionally had responsibility for alcohol education will, if encouraged to do so, gladly attend institutes on alcohol problems. But since these teachers usually have low status in faculty society, they can be expected to accomplish little in the way of changing the school's climate. It would be far better to persuade some of the most influential members of the faculty, regardless of their fields or prior interest in alcohol problems, to attend such an institute. The school principal could use personal appeals and other, more tangible inducements, and he could promise his faculty members a most interesting experience. He might, indeed, decide to go himself.

Educational Procedures

Many authorities agree that group discussion is the best procedure in alcohol education. The teacher must be a discussion leader, seeing to it that all points of view are attended to, that minority views are respected, that all the students participate, and that objectivity and fair-mindedness are maintained.

When alcohol and drinking are discussed in an atmosphere of frankness and mutual confidence, other issues—particularly moral issues of a more general sort—will inevitably be raised, for, as we have seen, alcohol problems are embedded in a context of more general attitudes and values. By the same token, a discussion that starts with attention to family relations or school social life or rules and their enforcement will very likely get around to drinking. Most important for the students' development is what is "caught" from the teacher rather than what is "taught," and it is precisely on such "catching" occasions that students are most receptive to the facts that the teacher is able to present.

There are many settings, both formal and informal, in which discussion of this kind can take place. It should not be assumed that alcohol education belongs only to the "problems" courses; rather, all teachers, whatever their courses, should sense when it is appropriate to "get off the subject" and have a free discussion of whatever concerns the students.

The best time to offer the most important lessons about alcohol and drinking is when crises around these subjects have arisen in the school: for example, when there has been a large-scale infringement of school rules or state law. At such times there is no problem about getting the students' attention. Students may use these occasions to test whether their teachers are prepared to listen and to be honest. Much depends on whether or not this test is passed.

For some students, it does not take a school crisis or a sensational news story to arouse interest in or concern about alcohol and drinking. These students usually already have problems; for example, one may have a parent or close relative who is a problem drinker, another may have strong religious or moral reasons for not drinking but is under strong social pressure to drink, a third may be worried about his own drinking. There must be adults to whom these young people can talk. Here a measure of specialized knowledge, not only of how to relate to young people, but of alcohol problems is called for, either on the part of professional counselors or student-oriented teachers who have informed themselves in some depth.

Readiness for alcohol education can be induced. Probably the best way is to combine education with inquiry. For example, samples of students might be interviewed for research purposes and then offered feedback in discussion groups. Also, students themselves can take part in investigations; for example, as junior members of research teams, they could help to collect data at their own schools. Those who become "authorities" in this manner could be expected to teach others, and their "findings" would spread throughout the school.

The lecture and other didactic procedures are not to be altogether despised. It is well known that some students prefer these procedures and learn more from them than they do from free discussions. There are places for formal presentations of material about alcohol and drinking, and these places—the best ones—are within a series or within a context of similar phenomena or related problems, as in a social-science or mental-hygiene course or in a series of lectures on campus problems. Single lectures on alcohol problems by outside speakers invited by school authorities should, as a rule, be avoided. Not only would most students stay away, but the lecture, as a "special event," would tend to confirm the special and specially ambivalent way in which these problems tend to be regarded.

Curriculum

However much we may accent attitudes, motivation for learning, and the general climate of the school, the fact remains that there is "content" to be learned: facts and principles about alcohol and drinking that should have a place in the school curriculum. Those interested in alcohol education should not, however, engage in competition with other interest groups for classroom hours, space in textbooks, and so on. Instead, there should be continuing efforts to integrate alcohol-related phenomena with the general curriculum, both with subjects in the "education for living" area and with traditional academic subjects.

Educators concerned with helping students to understand their contemporary environment and to deal with the problems it poses should search for common ground, for ways of relating their interests, for general principles that govern the particular problematic phenomena. For example, some aspects of alcohol education are natural parts of driver education; alcohol and drugs of various kinds may for some purposes be discussed together; and drinking behavior can be regarded as a special case of impulse expression.

More important than finding for alcohol and drinking an integral place in the "education for living" area is the task of showing students and faculty that alcohol problems are intellectually challenging and worthy of study in various scientific and humanistic contexts. It must be shown, indeed, that the study of alcohol problems may help to advance understanding in various subject areas.

In biology, for example, the problem of alcoholism can be used to bring students quickly to the frontiers of knowledge, to show that much remains for *them* eventually to find out. Although alcohol metabolism is well understood as a very special case of metabolism in general, the question of what happens in the body, particularly in the brain, as a result of prolonged exposure to alcohol remains unanswered. Biology teachers have here an excellent opportunity to show how their science deals with a mystery.

Teachers of history might well give attention to the "noble experiment," prohibition, as a means for revealing major trends in the American ethos and for showing something of how our political system works. By explaining why it is that in Western stories and movies Indians become roaring drunk after imbibing a little "firewater," while cowboys and settlers become better shots the more they drink, they can make some nice points about American culture and about ethnocentrism. By explaining how the repeal of prohibition was brought off, they can teach how existing laws about alcohol might be improved.

In courses in literature, teachers will need only to call attention to the matter in order to have students learn through their reading something of the diversity of group drinking practices in different times and places, and something of the various meanings that drinking may have for the individual. The teacher may use literary accounts of drinking to serve various purposes, for example, to give lessons in the relativity of values, or, by showing the wide range of human motives and feelings, to help students to be more accepting of themselves—a basic requirement for integrative drinking or for abstaining.

PREVENTION THROUGH A BROAD-BASED COMMUNITY EFFORT

Legislative hearings on lowering the legal age for drinking would be a good occasion for discussion in the popular press of issues concerning the role of youth in our society, the conditions that favor individual development, the problem of freedom and responsibility, and so on. This proposed change in the law would immediately create interesting problems for discussion on college campuses, for colleges and universities would have to take up immediately the issue of reviewing their own rules. This would be a great opportunity to confront these institutions with the question of how to promote integrative drinking. It would not be difficult to make clear to these institutions that just changing their rules without taking advantage of the situation to promote educational objectives would be to miss a great opportunity. This would be the time and the place to urge not only that patterns of campus drinking should be such as to favor the individual student's integrating his drinking within his personality structure, but that this institution might utilize drinking practices in the interests of its own strivings to become more of a community. Thus, for example, special efforts should be made to see to it that the campus pub or rathskeller become a meeting place for both students and faculty so that at last a way would have been found to bring these two groups together, in nonacademic settings, in ways that favor their genuine acquaintanceship.

As Wilkinson (in press) has suggested, any kind of action involving a change of existing laws or a fresh effort at public enlightenment about alcohol should, if possible, be carried out with the cooperation of the liquor industry. Lowering the drinking age would open up for the industry a new market, and we should expect a flood of advertising directed to this market. Here it would be a fine thing, for example, if advertising depicted older and younger people, such as students and faculty, drinking together, and it would also be a fine thing if such advertising, at the same time, suggested that the abstainer also exists in our society and has every right to his freedom of choice. The point being made here is that there should be an interaction between legal or administrative actions on the one hand and educational activities or activities aimed at public enlightenment on the other. The same kind of consideration would hold for a proposal for laws that would help to institute family drinking places. Such a proposal would once again arouse public interest and create opportunities for putting across enlightened views. By the same token, proposed innovations for alcohol education in the schools might easily arouse concern, if not opposition, among parents. This response should be regarded not as blocking by parents of a progressive measure but as an opportunity to educate parents at the same time their children are educated.

It goes without saying that any proposal to lower the drinking age should be accompanied by a proposal that greater strictness be exercised in controlling the drinking of high-school youth. Indeed, any argument for lowering the drinking age has to be based in a developmental theory which states that by the age of 18, on the average, the ego is sufficiently well developed so that drinking may become integrative. This is essentially the same developmental theory that may be used as a basis for saying that people younger than 18 (to strike an average) ought to wait. Propositions of this kind have enormous implications for programs of alcohol education in the schools, and the point being made here is that what is done in the schools cannot be separated from what is done in the larger society, and that what is done by legal means cannot be separated from what is done through efforts at public enlightenment.

REFERENCES

Cooperative Commission on the Study of Alcoholism. *Alcohol problems: a report to the nation.* New York: Oxford Univer. Press, 1967.

Fallding, H. The source and burden of civilization illustrated in use of alcohol. *Quart. J. Stud. Alcohol.*, 1964, **25**, 714-724.

Wilkinson, R. *The prevention of drinking problems.* New York: Oxford Univer. Press, in press.

III

APPROACHES
TO RESEARCH
AND ACTION

Concern with a value base and with a particular theoretical orientation also underlies or characterizes the five chapters in this part. They address themselves more specifically, however, to research and action in particular community systems—the city and the neighborhood—and to describing particular approaches to the solution of system and social problems— the T group, the self-help group or organization, and training in new careers.

Chapter 10 gives a comprehensive overview of approaches to research in the urban environment. After presenting a number of perspectives from which the city can be viewed—as a bureaucracy, as a place in time, as an economic entity, and as a system— the authors go on to discuss conditions for successful urban problem solving and suggest a set of approaches through which behavioral science can be used as a scientific base for urban decision making. Of particular interest is the fact that this is not a "tourist" view, but a participant conceptualization from the vantage point of both the university and the central administrative office of one of the world's largest cities.

From concern with the total city, the focus moves to one neighborhood, in the contribution by Rhodes, Seeman, Spielberger, and Stepbach. Chapter 11 provides an example of the integration of theory, practice, and research in an interdisciplinary project which serves as a bridge from the university to the community, providing at the same time an opportunity for training in community psychology. Because both its practice and research appear to be firmly grounded in sociological and psychological theory as well as in community-organization principles, this kind of center may well become a core model for the community psychologist action-researcher-teacher.

The city and the neighborhood are two of the major systems within which the community psychologist works. He has moved from behind his desk into the community, and with this move has come the development of new methods and techniques.

Noting the wide discrepancy between democratic belief and actual practice in the schools, Hassol describes the use of a "sensitivity group" democratic approach in helping resolve intergroup and intragroup problems. Chapter 12 provides a vivid illustration of the effectiveness of this technique and discusses its broader significance for the educational system and for communication between the generations. It also implicitly raises an issue initially raised by Rhodes, in Chapter 2. In the relationship between the community and the "deviant" individual, to what extent should there be an attempt to change the individual to fit in with community expectations? To what extent should there be an attempt to change community attitudes toward greater acceptance of the individual?

The subtitle of Chapter 13, on Synanon, by Enright is appropriately "A Challenge to Middle-Class Views of Mental Health." It describes the broadening of the Synanon base to work with many kinds of people in innovative ways. The game clubs described in this chapter might be viewed as one of a spectrum of group developments on the current scene. Certainly, community psychologists need to be aware of these developments and to consider the meaning of their widespread acceptance and the challenge they present to traditional views and approaches.

The final chapter in this part, by the Grants, provides still another example of the use of a group approach, this time in the context of research and as a method for training in new careers. The community-psychology educator might well note the outline of group activities used in training for new careers: study groups in research methods, in interviewing techniques, in group dynamics, and in organization change, among others. Insofar as the "new careers" movement is based on an education and not on a therapy model, it might be said to epitomize the "growth and development" emphases of community psychology.

CHAPTER 10

Cities, Behavioral Research, and Community Mental Health

Timothy W. Costello and Sheldon S. Zalkind

Two out of every three Americans live in one of the country's twenty major cities, or in an area dominated by one (Gruen, 1964). No one can know very much about America unless he knows what is happening in its cities, nor can anyone plan for improvements in the quality of life and health in America without working through its large urban complexes.

Many of our urban problems can be viewed as symptoms of community mental-health problems, as sources of high stress that increase the probability of psychological disorders, or as barriers to dealing with mental-health problems (or, of course, all three). Hollingshead and Redlich (1958), among others, have shown some of the relationships of socioeconomic level to the incidence and treatment of behavior disorders.

This chapter attempts to describe approaches to urban problems, drawn from the less clinical areas of psychology and the other behavioral sciences, that are relevant to community mental health but different from the other useful community mental-health concerns presented elsewhere in this book. We propose here to lay out for a readership in community mental health:

1. Ways of thinking about cities.

2. Some conditions for successful urban problem solving.

3. Behavioral-science research approaches that might be helpful.

4. Two examples of the approaches described: one, a synthesizing of some research on aggression; and the other, an illustration

of an experimental approach to a community problem.

We hope that our approach can serve as one framework within which the more specialized and technical approaches described elsewhere in the book can be applied. Such application should both take account of the highly complex nature of urban society and its influence on the individual and, as well, fully utilize the resources of the several behavioral sciences.

WAYS OF THINKING ABOUT CITIES

The community mental-health program can be developed and related to the city within the perspective of any of five different ways of thinking about cities. Mental-health workers may need to deal with people who view a city, sometimes only implicitly, from one or another of these perspectives. And the community mental-health program itself may have to be examined from each of these viewpoints to get at the variety of factors that are relevant to its aims.

As a Bureaucracy

If one focuses on its managing processes, the city can be described as a bureaucracy. It is run by a growing number of civil servants, arranged in careful hierarchical relation to each other and well trained to know and apply highly specific rules governing the allocation of municipal resources: money, land use, privilege, and influence. When viewed as a bureaucracy, the city's principal characteristic is its capacity to maintain the status quo as it preserves the reward-distributing patterns of the past and interprets rules designed to implement goals previously established. Advantages of the city's existence as a bureaucracy are the orderliness and predictability of its behavior and its capacity to keep large numbers of people (300,000 in New York City) employed in stable and related ways. In a rapidly changing society, the disadvantages are important: inflexibility, slowness of response, exclusion of new ideas and new people, and a tendency to see rule enforcement as an end in itself, to the detriment of effective problem solving.

Directors of community mental-health programs need to know how to operate within their municipal bureaucracy while, at the same time, members of their staffs may be working to reduce its bureaucratic rigidities.

As a Place in Space and Time

But the city is also a physical entity. It may be placed at the juncture of three state lines, sprawled across a number of islands, or stretched along the border of a neighboring county. It may be cut up by railroad lines coming in from all points of the compass. Some cities are dominated by their large, useful harbors; others by their being centered in mining, cattle, or agricultural country. Temperature and rainfall are important characteristics.

Technological advances having reduced the importance of geographical factors and man's well-known capacity for adjusting to a wide range of environments make this way of thinking about a city less valuable than it formerly was. But it cannot be disregarded. Geographical characteristics influence available work opportunities, affect the flow of in-migration, raise or lower the cost of living, and limit or expand recreational and leisure-time activities.

Often, the historical factors that initiated a city's growth continue to operate and affect its style of living and the nature of its problems. The motion-picture industry of Los Angeles; the slaughterhouses of Chicago; the garment industry, strong union movement, and immigration patterns of New York; the dominant universities of Boston—all continue to shape their cities in different ways. Mental-health problems are different at least in subtle ways, because of the different developmental histories of the cities in which they occur. Mental-health programs must, therefore, be tuned in to the special historical characteristics of the cities in which they operate.

Even more directly related to mental health are the characteristics of a city that the anthropologist describes. Most large cities show great similarity in the ways their people deal with everyday problems of living. Nevertheless, significant differences do exist. Despite gross similarities, Harlem is not Watts; Harlem differs even from neighboring Bedford-Stuyvesant and the South Bronx. The ways family members help each other, religious beliefs and practices, child-rearing practices, attitudes toward old age are not primarily determined by the city (or even community) of residence; yet the different geographical and historical characteristics of cities do have important effects on these aspects of human behavior. Within cities, distinctive communal and family behavior can provide both mental-health strengths and weaknesses.

As a Political Entity

No mental-health worker—whose funds are dependent on national, state, and local legislatures and whose freedom to act is dependent on laws and administrative interpretations—is likely to be unaware of the importance of politics. But here we speak of the city itself, whose boundaries contain the urban mental-health program, as a political entity. Cities are creatures of the state, with more or less home rule. Of all levels of government, they suffer the most extensive set of political constraints. They are dominated by the meanest level of political power and are subject to the most obstreperous pressure groups. Municipal government is bound into entangling alliances and coalitions, requiring continual bargain and compromise. Political-party membership is important, and elections and electioneering are dominating concerns. There is always the possibility of scandal and corruption.

From this mare's nest, most mental-health workers would wish to be delivered. Sadly, we argue, they cannot be above politics; they should be right in the middle of it, constituting one of the pressure blocs, hobnobbing with public officials, battling to maintain and raise the status of their program, lobbying for better legislation, more money, and greater freedom to act. The community's attitude toward mental health, for good or for bad, may depend on the quality of politicking engaged in by their mental-health leaders.

As an Economic Entity

At some level of analysis, a city's mental-health program is a percentage of the gross urban product. It is so many dollars paid in fees or allocated out of tax dollars. On the other side, the program can be added up as salaries and rent paid, maintenance and operating costs. From this point of view, the mental-health leader must take account of the city as an economic entity.

New York City's budget of $6.2 billion is next in size to the federal government's. What percentage of that budget is allocated to mental health; what would be an ideal figure? What estimates of the cost effectiveness of various mental-health programs are available to argue the case? What is the relation between unemployment rates and demands for mental-health services? Between minimum-wage level and such services? How can the tax base be increased to provide more funds? What kind of tax program is fairest and best from a mental-health point of view? Do major industries provide stable employment and salary levels? Is the rate of economic activity moving up or down?

There are no Rorschach indices to provide answers for any of these questions. No usual three-discipline conference spends much time on them. Yet there are mental-health implications in all the questions. For that reason we are persuaded that the mental-health program must reach into the economic sector, gathering information and effecting change. The city's economy is an aspect of its mental health.

As a System

Granted that a city manages its affairs through its huge bureaucracy, exists in a particular place, has a unique history, is very much involved in politics, and faces enormous economic problems, anyone who has ever tried to do anything about a city's problems knows that it is, above all, a huge and complex set of intricately interrelated activities, processes, and structures. It is, in the technical sense of the term, a *system*, although it is to all appearances anything but "systematic" (in another use of the word) in its behavior. Looking at the city as a system is undoubtedly the most helpful viewpoint, whether the viewer is a mental-health worker, a sanitation engineer, a commissioner of welfare, or a concerned citizen. A systems approach includes the other viewpoints already described. It highlights the fact that everything about a city affects everything else in the city: that change in one area is both dependent upon and a definite influence on all other areas; that any urban process is only one line of tension tied into a network of tensions; that any structure is supported by building blocks of all the other structures. In a system as large and complex as a city, the interrelatedness of the almost infinite number of parts makes for inertia, frustration, and a sense of being overwhelmed by the difficulties of accomplishing anything at all. But there is a positive side: successfully cleaning up one city street, just because everything is related to everything else, will make it easier to clean up others.

Working one mental-health program through the bureaucracy and political pressure groups can have beneficial effects on other parts of the system. In any system, solving one problem, even a small one, makes it easier to work on other problems.

Aside from the factor of interrelatedness, a systems point of view offers other interesting ways of approaching urban problems. Different models can be used. For example, the city can be usefully conceptualized as a biological system, and its problems analyzed in terms of biological structures and processes. The human nervous system can serve as a model for analyzing communications and decision-making problems. Problems of air, water, and street pollution can usefully be seen as aspects of a unitary metabolic process. Forces maintaining or disturbing the city's homeostatic balance can be identified. Concepts of growth, maturity, and decay can be applied to cities as a whole or to their constituent communities. The biological model can provide some different ways of thinking about community mental health. A community is healthy when its biological processes are normally functioning: a criterion for assessing the impact of a mental-health program might be the cleanness of its community streets, or the swiftness and accuracy with which its nervous system handles information.

Still within the systems point of view, a variant of the biological model is the behavioral-science model. Cities and communities "behave": they perceive events, are subject to motivational influences, learn, and respond with emotion. Mental-health questions, particularly, can be cast in terms of municipal or community behavior patterns: For example, what are the characteristics of the community's perceptual apparatus? How does distortion take place? How can distortion be reduced? We will consider the behavioral-sciences model in further detail later in the chapter.

SOME CONDITIONS FOR SUCCESSFUL URBAN PROBLEM SOLVING [1]

Presidents, mayors, citizens, and social scientists have identified and described the problems of our large cities. The problems are severe and many, and community mental-health programs come into immediate contact with them.

New York City's problems, although many times larger in scope,

[1]This section and the one following ("Behavioral-Science Approaches") have been adapted from Costello and Zalkind (1968).

are illustrative of problems that perplex Chicago, Detroit, Boston, and other cities. In New York, one-third of the students who enter high school drop out before graduation. Among minority ethnic groups, increasingly becoming the core groups in large cities, unemployment is twice the national rate. For young Negroes and Puerto Ricans, unemployment is four times the national rate. The bulk of the severe narcotics problems is centered in a half-dozen large cities; perhaps half the problem resides in New York City, where there are 100,000 addicts. Crime increases at a rate beyond the containment capacity of any rehabilitative process. New York City's rate jumped 14 per cent in one year (not attributable to new record keeping). As to congestion: 100,000 families (all of them living in inadequate congested slums) are on a waiting list for public housing. The wait is frequently longer than two years. Many other families and individuals are so crushed that they lack the energy to make application or are excluded from applying by the social criteria used in selection.

Each of the major urban problems both feeds on and feeds into all the other problems. School dropouts have difficulty finding employment. Long periods of unemployment lead to escapist and defensive behavior—drug addiction and crime. To complete the cycle, the unstable family life that results increases the likelihood of school failure. Bad housing increases the probability of maladjusted behavior, but unsocialized families run down decent housing. The intricate and deplorable system goes on endlessly; it seems almost impossible to enter it at any point to reverse its direction.

A massive approach, attacking the whole system all at once, is required. And this is what the federal model-cities legislation proposes. The difficulties of implementing the legislation are immense, and the tools available to municipalities are grossly inadequate.

What is required to develop a systems approach to urban problems described? It seems to us there are five essential conditions:

1. A stable community power structure.
2. Adequate fiscal resources.
3. Flexible and dependable federal legislation.
4. A civil-service work force that is both skilled and motivated.
5. A political base that is regional, not narrowly local.

None of these conditions prevail in most of the large cities in the United States.

A Stable Community Power Structure

Accepting Bertrand Russell's definition of *power* as "the production of intended effects" (Russell, 1962), we point out that a mayor of a large city does not have, by himself or in his government, the power to achieve his goals in all the sectors and communities of his city. What he needs is access to those individuals and groups (the Establishment) who do have power among their own constituencies (the multiple constituencies adding up to the whole city). But the old Establishment has been badly shaken, and its power weakened. No stable power elite has yet taken its place. In New York City there is no one to talk to who has the power in Harlem or in the South Bronx or the North Bronx for that matter. As a result, there is endless dickering, conflict, and inaction. The model-cities program is caught in a morass of conflicting demands; poverty programs pit one group against another; within school districts the "community" has various voices speaking for it. The sine qua non for systematic, orderly change in a large organization, a stable hierarchy of power relations, is absent in our large cities because power itself is changing hands.

Adequate Fiscal Resources

The Ribicoff Committee on Governmental Reorganization suggested that $50 billion was required to make a beginning on only one urban problem, housing. A barely perceptible fraction of that sum has been made available in dribs and drabs of often unrelated legislation. The cities themselves do not have access to the money that is required. Urban problems do not develop in relation to revenue-producing possibilities. The number of families on welfare in a city is unrelated to the local rate of economic activity, and may be more related to agricultural technology and to the way welfare legislation is written in other parts of the nation. Tenements must be replaced, but this cannot be done at a profit, nor does it produce increased taxes. A reduction in school dropouts does not increase gross city product for many years to come. Programs to solve urban problems are not self-liquidating. The required subsidies cannot be found in the meager tax sources not pre-empted by federal and state law. Solutions to urban problems have to be subsidized with federal funds, and no adequate sum of dollars has been provided.

The movement now is to use federal funds as seed money to attract dollars from the private sector. Programs are being discussed—one or two are already in operation—that will provide tax rebates, training funds, or federal insurance. The idea is promising, but it is untested and a long way from implementation.

Flexible and Dependable Federal Legislation

"Not enough" is only one complaint that cities have about what comes from Washington. What comes is not dependable and/or too rigidly imposed. Funds are allocated on an annual basis, making impossible the long-range and stable planning that is required for maximum impact on the problems. Many programs are set up on a demonstration basis: established for a year and then cut off from federal support. Frequent changes in federal legislation or changing administrative interpretations impose shifting policies and reversed decisions on municipalities, so that whatever good is done is often undone. The legislation, at least in the past, has been written with so many restraints in it as to make impossible the flexible use of the funds provided as circumstances vary from one city to another and from one time period to another.

A Skilled and Motivated Civil Service

Bases of power in the community and adequate federal funds flexibly and dependably provided are required, but, at bottom, the municipal job is performed by employees—professional, technical, administrative—in the civil service. The long, important shadow of a mayor is the work done by career public servants—selected, trained, and rewarded under a merit system in accord with civil-service law. Many of us on the urban front are considering whether that law isn't now preventing what it was set up to assure—a high-quality, well-motivated work force in public service. Merit defined as a score on a test, tenure granted as lifetime security in a particular job, reward given as a mandated salary increase once or twice a year—these neither attract ability nor motivate performance.

While the civil-service law may still serve to reduce political or personal favoritism and to attract some job applications, in most large cities it has become a rigid protective device for maintaining the status quo. It has allowed employees to become frozen to past procedures and practices, impervious to influence by policy changes at the top. The problem among employees is not the lack of talent or of capacity to be motivated. It is the system that hampers talent and disengages the energies of the employee from the influence efforts of the manager. Recent growth in union membership among public employees has only intensified the difficulties. Union muscle is now an additional force used on management to maintain what was, and union leadership is seen by many employees to have more effect on the reward system than a man's own boss.

A Regional Political Base

There is, finally, the question of whether or not cities have adequate governmental scope to command the resources needed to solve their problems. Again using New York City as an example, we can show that for two reasons the conditions of adequate governmental power are not met. The governmental base of New York is its five boroughs in which some 8 million people live. It is surrounded by more than 50 political entities, all independent of New York, whose 8–9 million people profit, in one way or another, from being close to New York and whose activities, in one way or another, add to the problems, fiscal and others, of the city. The city has limited means of taxing the outside group (Mayor Lindsay's commuter tax was a minimal breakthrough) or of affecting their actions. There is, in other words, a lack of correspondence between the resource base and the service base. Comparable situations exist in other large cities surrounded by politically independent suburban communities.

There is a second weakness in the political base of the large cities. Congressional and legislative apportionment continues to favor the less populated areas of the country. Voting behavior reflects that distribution to the disadvantage of the large metropolitan complexes, as well as the cities. Federal and, frequently, state allocations are made in ways that do not totally match the distribution of problems between urban and nonurban areas.

BEHAVIORAL-SCIENCE APPROACHES

The nation's cities are facing formidable problems under conditions that handicap problem-solving efforts. To a considerable extent, political action is required to change the conditions. But that action will not come soon. It will certainly not come all at once. To work within the reality of the adverse conditions described, with any hope of making progress, urban managers need to be given as much of a scientific base as is possible for their decisions. Much of that base, in our judgment, must be drawn from behavioral science.

Particularly if a systems approach is to be taken to urban problems, there must be a systematic effort to organize scientific resources—research methods as well as research findings—into an urban framework. The contributions of the behavioral sciences to the solution of urban problems can come from both the implications of already existing collections of information concerning human behavior and the adaption to urban problems of behavioral-research methods. Therefore, we turn now from the problems themselves to a description of a set of approaches through which behavioral science can be used to provide some scientific foundation for urban decision making. We believe that community mental-health workers are already utilizing some of these approaches.

Comparative Approaches

A good way to begin is to recognize that cities are different, one from another—different not only in location, size, and citizenry, but also in their history of successes and failures and in their respective performance levels. We haven't learned how to take advantage of these differences to improve our methods for solving problems. We talk of cities as if their housing problems, school problems, race problems, and so on were as alike in nature as they are in label; as if the cities were all doing about the same things to solve their problems; and, finally, as if the cities were all equally successful or unsuccessful.

There are many specific and important differences among cities, despite the common labeling of their problems. Last summer some cities had riots and others did not. Where there were riots, reactions varied from city to city. There are differences in the degree to which cities have been able to capture federal aid: if New York had as much federal aid per capita as New Haven or even Boston, the allocation would exhaust the entire federal budget available for urban aid. Focus of effort is different: the urbanists of Los Angeles are spending their energies in different ways from the urbanists of New York; and Chicago's effort might be different from both.

These and other differences provide useful data for comparative studies of cities. Paul Lazarsfeld (1959), years ago, pointed out that behavioral scientists must use organizations as if each were a unit in the total sample. Organizational psychologists have since done so with insightful results. We should begin to do the same with cities, so that the unit of observation is a city among a sample of cities. Conclusions can then be drawn from a sample of ten or twenty cities, varied in size and location. Blanche Blank (1966) has expressed the idea that cities be compared on total-city performance, with comparisons that could be international in scope.

Riecken (1966), in a summary for the Social Science Research Council, describes five approaches to a comparative sociology across cultures. His approaches, it seems to us, could be usefully applied to intercity comparisons.

The Classical Dependent-Variable Approach. In the field of urban research, where experience is scant and control difficult, it may be permitted to work in a direction the reverse of the usual experimental approach, that is, to go from dependent to independent variable. Thus, the first step is to identify urban outputs in which cities are likely to vary. The second step is to work backward to identify possible independent variables that might account for the differences in outputs. As a simple illustration, group together five cities that had riots and five that did not. What else is similar or different between the two groups? Or take the rates of unemployment among minority populations of ten cities where those rates were different, and consider that the dependent variable or criterion. Arrange the cities into two groups, high and low; then identify other differences among the cities. Where relationships seem to exist, useful hypotheses might develop that could be subjected to more rigorous testing.

The Total-City Approach. A profile could be developed for each of a number of major cities, using dimensions that at least in the beginning might be selected on the basis of informed guesses about which are significant. The profile should include a description of each city's geography, its relation to oceans and rivers, its means of transportation, its climate, ethnic balance, stability of population, migration trends, and industries. Several profiles might be developed that would define each city uniquely along significant dimensions. Once the profiles are developed, they could be studied in relation to various outputs of each city: the occurrence of riots, performance measures, pace of integration, quality of education, and so on.

The Narrow Entering-Wedge Approach. With this approach, we select some highly specific event or process that has taken place in a number of cities and use this as a point of departure to understand causal relations between the event and a variety of other factors. For example, some 200 cities submitted applications for model-cities grants. It might be worthwhile to use that fact as an entering wedge for an exploration of how different cities behave and what happens as a result. How did cities write their applications? Who was used to help—"in-house" talent, consultants, scientists, what categories of scientists? How did the products differ? Which kinds were successful in receiving funds? What resulted in the urban communities during the process and afterward? If our longitudinal effort is maintained for a sufficient period of time, we might even discover which processes resulted in the building of model cities and which did not and why not.

The Behavioral-Science Concept. Riecken suggests that it is useful to take a well-developed concept in the behavioral sciences and study various cultures (in our case cities) in relation to it. One that comes to mind is the concept of participation, which is, in the twentieth century, almost platitudinous, yet not at all a target of research in urban settings. There are different ways of achieving "maximum feasible participation." How do cities vary in their approaches? What are the characteristics of cities where participation has been extensive? How do they differ from other cities? Have the effects of participation been different for cities with different characteristics? Was there more participation in cities without riots? Or was it the other way? Data to answer these questions, we believe, exist but have not yet been mined.

The Experimental Approach. With cities as units, control and experimental groups can be set up to test in more precise fashion the relationships between independent and dependent variables. The opportunities for experimental manipulations on cities are not many, but they can be found. We can suggest a realistic example: the urban summer program, in which employment for thousands of teenagers, particularly from minority groups, is provided. There are two ways of funding the summer program, publicly or privately. Much more is involved than where the money comes from, however; there are differences between the two methods in selection, training, types of jobs, supervision, controls, and future opportunities. At the moment, we have no research to say which method (granted the equal availability of both) has the better effect. With a little imagination and entrepreneurship, both intracity and intercity experiments could be run. There are other problems: clean-up campaigns, for example, where the effects of different plans could be studied in loose, experimental fashion among a sample of comparable communities. (A more detailed example of the experimental approach is presented later in the chapter.)

It must be obvious to the reader that the comparative urban studies we are talking about go beyond superficial exchanges among cities on current practices. Information about municipal practices is regularly exchanged; there are slick magazines that survive by promoting such informational exchanges. We are talking about a rigorous research program conducted over a long period of time with strong scientific controls.

Other Research Approaches

Concurrently, and with some hope of more immediate gains, other research approaches can be developed. We describe three briefly.

The Synthesizing Approach. There is a great body of behavioral research already done. Berelson and Steiner (1964) have summarized basic aspects of it conveniently. What is needed is to comb out of this literature the research relevant to urban programs and to synthesize it in a form that would be helpful to urban decision makers.

Two examples illustrate the suggestion. As previously mentioned, many cities have summer programs during which thousands of teenagers are given summer employment. Aside from the fact that it seems a worthwhile activity and that keeping teenagers busy and off the streets is a way to "cool" the summer, the program doesn't have any specific goals. Yet there is a body of research on level of aspiration, need achievement, and role development that could be useful in making the program more than an interim way of avoiding trouble. Selection, training, work experiences, and supervision could be planned to raise levels of aspiration, strengthen need achievement and motivation, and build role identifications if appropriate research findings were delivered to the proper people at the proper time. Here is a contribution to be made by some behavioral scientists who will summarize the research in the context of this urban problem.

Another example can be drawn from the federal mandate to achieve "maximum feasible participation" from community groups. There is extensive research on participation, although there is little on specific urban applications. Extrapolation from nonurban problems should be allowed under the circumstances.[2] What does the research tell us about maximizing willingness to allow participation or to gain acceptance of an invitation to participate (for example, only 1 per cent of the poverty population may actually vote in community elections)? How can participation by target populations also allow counsel by experts? What types of problems are best dealt with through participative interaction? The questions ask a lot from behavioral research. But at the moment they are being answered on the urban scene largely without benefit of any significant data. (The synthesizing approach is also illustrated more fully later in the chapter.)

The Model Approach. Can a city be viewed as a biosocial organism and be better understood by analyzing its life processes? Wolman (1965) has written about sanitation, air and water pollution as aspects of the city's metabolic processes. Are there not in the city also perceptual, motivational, learning, and attitudinal processes that can be analyzed in relation to urban problems and to behavioral-science research? We don't want to speak of a collective mind. But it does seem possible to identify characteristics of an urban perceptual apparatus and helpful to study that apparatus in relation to what we have discovered about the perceptual process generally. The reward systems in cities—influence, land use, tax assessments, and privileges—underlie the dynamics of urban life.

[2]Here, as elsewhere, a synthesizer must watch for the shifting use of terminology. An experiment often distinguishes between "participation" and "representation" and shows the results to be different. The urban problem solver who has invited community "participation"—but has "representation"—might have confused expectations as to the outcome.

How can they be conceptualized as a motivational process? Cities, as social organizations, learn, and the urban learning process can be analyzed. We believe ways can be found of helping urbanists by conceiving of the city as an organic whole and filling in the bits and pieces of social-science research that relate to the social and psychological processes of that organism.

The Problem-Oriented Approach. Perhaps the simplest, most direct approach, with the earliest payoff, is to begin with a problem cities have and ask behavioral scientists how they would solve it. For example, what are the best ways of resolving (managing) conflict? in the labor-relations field? between community groups? among political leaders? What is the best way to teach low-income people good consumer practices? How do you change attitudes of long-time public servants? of middle-class community groups? How—to be very daring—do you prevent riots?

Under this heading, the most important question is, without doubt, How do you get public officials to listen to behavioral scientists? This question points up the real issue we have raised: behavioral scientists and urbanists (municipal officials) each have much to gain by extensive cooperation. Producing that cooperation is a proper goal for the field of community mental health.

TWO RESEARCH APPROACHES ILLUSTRATED

We want now to elaborate more fully two research approaches referred to earlier, the synthesizing approach and the experimental approach. We claim no originality for the concepts discussed. Our goal is to relate well-known research findings and scientific methodology to urban problem-solving efforts.

A Synthesizing Approach: Examining Hate and Violence

Earlier in the chapter, we described a "synthesizing approach" in applying behavioral-science research to urban problems. There we sketchily illustrated that approach in the area of summer employment for teenagers and programs for community participation. Here we illustrate the approach more fully, using the problem of hate and violence.

The point we want to make needs to be stated precisely. Few people today question that "hate and violence" is the country's foremost domestic problem (if not also its prime international problem). At all levels of government, officials are taking action to "solve" the problem. Solutions are sought in many directions: changing the style of police response, using the National Guard, instituting urban-renewal programs, developing employment programs, using community leadership, encouraging more frequent interaction between ghetto communities and public officials. There may be merit in all the solutions sought, but rarely can public officials find a convenient, authoritative, and understandable summary of the abundant behavioral-science research done in the area so that they can use the findings to develop new programs and test existing programs against scientific findings. The same statement could be made about many other urban problems. The conclusions *not* to draw here are (1) that if such a summary were available, it would reveal sure solutions to the problems and (2) that the summary would, in the first instance, be read and, in the second, followed by the officials whose responsibility it is to take action on the problems. Conclusions that we *can* draw are (1) that behavioral-science research is relevant and useful to public officials and (2) that behavioral scientists have a responsibility to make that research available and to press for its consideration (along with other points of view) in decisions that are made. Community mental-health workers share that responsibility in the over-all sense and, in addition, have particular responsibility in their own community work.

Although newspapers and public reports use the terms *hate* and *violence*, our analysis speaks most often of *aggression*, because this is the term used in behavioral-science literature. We trust the difference is only a semantic one. The discussion that follows is meant only to suggest in one area the kinds of behavioral research that are directly relevant to urban problem solving. It is not at all offered as a definitive or comprehensive survey of the research that has been done. Our presentation focuses mostly on data from psychological research. The other behavioral sciences, of course, have much to contribute to an understanding of the problem.

Hate and violence are often found together, although each can occur independently of the other. Moynihan (1958) has put a new title on an old phenomenon. He speaks of "the new racialism," defining it as "racial prejudice or discrimination: race hatred," and he describes new expression of it in today's society. Present as an attitude in large numbers of both white and black citizens, prejudice or hate may exist for years, showing itself in a wide variety of discriminatory acts but not necessarily violence. Most whites who hate blacks, and blacks who hate whites, have developed social controls that keep aggression from being expressed.

Strangely enough, the opposite can also occur: violence without hate. Americans dropping bombs on Vietnam installations don't hate the people they kill. Catton (1953, pp. 172-173) writes about Confederate and Union soldiers swapping cigarettes across the battlelines, telling stories, and sharing family pictures, until the order to shoot was given, at which they all climbed back into their trenches and shot at each other. Strange behavior, indeed.

Hate and violence fall into different psychological categories. Hate is an attitude; violence must be expressed through overt behavior. But attitudes and behavior interact.

It is easy to understand that attitudes shape behavior, but the fact is that behavior also shapes attitudes. Hate pushes the individual toward aggressive and even violent behavior; but violence and aggression, once expressed, tend to build and support attitudes of hate toward their victims. It is this combination of hate and violence that sorely besets our cities today: blacks hating whites and rioting (or rioting and then hating whites), and whites hating blacks and beating them up (or discriminating actively against them for years and then hating them).

Today, hate and violence are seen not only in riots but also in the vitriolic campaigns of "impeach," "suppress," "censor" by so-called Freedom Forums attacking the patriotism of others. The hate may show, the violence may not. But the goal of destroying those holding opposing views is clear; there are deep-seated, ego-defensive, or ego-involved attitudes beng expressed. Everyone need not indulge in violence for the effects of their aggression to be seen. When mental-health and fluoridation programs are vehemently attacked as communist-inspired, when "law and order" slogans clearly imply ignoring due process of law, we are dealing with aggression.

There is behavioral-science research and theory on both attitudes and aggression that is relevant to the problem. Psychological factors that create and nourish attitudes have been identified, and attitude-changing procedures have been explored. The nature of aggression is still very much subject to debate, but some causes of aggressive behavior have been clearly identified and there are research-based suggestions for controlling it.

Hate. In this section, and in the one that follows, we accept the premise that changing attitudes or controlling behavior begins with our understanding the causes of each. We believe that we can better understand the development of hate by describing the functions of attitudes in general.

Attitudes develop and persist because they have value to the individual. Katz (1960, p. 254) identifies four functions that attitudes perform for the individual: (1) instrumental or utilitarian, (2) ego-defensive, (3) value-expressive, (4) knowledge. Following Katz, we suggest here how hate can be functional for the hater. The general theme is that *A* hates *B* (or all *B*'s) because it is satisfying for him to do so. To reduce or eliminate hate, we must deal with its motivational supports. Using Katz's four categories, we suggest the following possibilities:

1. Blacks hate whites because whites punish or thwart them (or, understandably, are perceived as doing so). To eliminate this motivational support for hate, whites must change their behavior and their image.

2. Some whites hate blacks because it protects their egos to do so. Other forms of ego defense (mental-hygiene approaches, for example) must be sought.

3. Blacks hate whites because it is part of their new identity to do so. Excising this element from a healthy new source of identity may be difficult but it is necessary.

4. Blacks and whites hate each other because it may be the only way for them to make sense of mixed-up society. Other answers must be carefully developed.

The social forces through which the functions of attitudes are developed and attitudes themselves are specified are the culture, the family-group memberships, and peer groups. If these groups serve as vehicles to carry people to socially undesired attitudes, they should be just as available for nullifying bad attitudes and arousing good ones. It is precisely here that community mental-health practice can and does make a major contribution to solving the problem. In addition, community mental-health workers and other behavioral scientists must make explicit for the public at large both the motivational bases of hate and the means available for changing attitudes.[3]

Aggression. Aggressive behavior appears so regularly throughout man's history and occurs so frequently in the behavior of most individuals that the conclusion is often drawn that aggression is an inevitable characteristic, an enduring and ineradicable aspect of human nature. Accepting it as such, some religions subsume it under original sin, Freudians consider it instinctual energy of the id, others regard it as one of man's basic attributes. While most behavioral scientists consider aggressive behavior an acquired or learned response (Montagu, 1968), the implication is often left that the learning of aggression is an inevitable part of man's adjustment to the world about him.

Whether or not man can create a world free from aggression is a question that cannot be answered on a scientific base to everyone's satisfaction. A less extreme proposition, we believe, can be supported in psychological theory: that aggressive behavior can be reduced and reshaped; that, in other words, something can be done to control it. Sufficient scientific study has been done on aggression to allow us to identify some of its causes. From that point, it is not impossible to plan a program of prevention.

For our limited purposes in this section, we describe five principal forms of aggression.[4]

1. Instrumental aggression. After the work of Thorndike, Skinner, and others more recently, no one questions that when behavior is followed (reinforced) by a satisfying state of affairs that behavior is more likely to recur. Assume a very simple situation: A child, taller or heavier than his peers, discovers that when he pushes a smaller child down, he gets what he wants; and a pattern of aggressive behavior is readily established. Where aggressive behavior is instrumental in goal achievement, it will become more frequent and more persistent. Examples more complex than the one we have used can readily be found in individual, group, and national behavior; the dynamics are the same.

We need to refer to two other principles from the field of operant conditioning[5] to understand more fully the learning of aggression as a response to reward. Human beings, particularly,

---

[3]A convenient summary of attitude-change procedures is in Katz (1960).

[4]Important sources here are Berkowitz (1962) and Scott (1958).

[5]The relevant principles of learning may be found summarized in many books, for example, Hilgard and Atkinson (1967).

generalize quickly from one situation to another. An individual (or group) finding aggression rewarded in one situation will generalize that response to other similar situations, and broad patterns of aggression are soon established. When it is also recalled that behavior rewarded sporadically or occasionally persists longer than behavior rewarded according to some pattern (after all rewards are withdrawn), one can easily see that society effectively teaches its members to be aggressive. The hopeful thing is that, knowing the rules of the game, we can just as effectively teach ourselves not to be aggressive.

In a general way, most people understand, as a matter of common sense, the ways in which rewards work to strengthen desired behavior. Unfortunately, for a variety of reasons, the knowledge is not applied. Sometimes, for example, the early expressions of violence or aggression are so threatening as to cause people (public officials, community authorities, or parents) to give in to demands out of fear. In New York City, the day after a group of young people rampaged through the civic area, destroying property and upsetting thousands of bystanders, the city announced an increase in funds for summer jobs—a desirable step but one that *seemed* to reward violence. Occasionally, the violence leads to rewards directly, for example, looting. It is understandable, therefore, that most people do not wish to reward rioters in their looting. Nevertheless, the rioting behavior needs to be understood as, at least partly, a response to the fact that over the years nonrioting, passive, or controlled behavior has not been rewarding to the groups now rioting.

There is another problem here. Sometimes what is known about rewards is just reversed and applied to punishment: If rewards strengthen certain responses, punishment will deter them. Research does not support so simple a conclusion. The effects of punishment are unpredictable (Costello & Zalkind, 1963, p. 215). In an urban context, punishment more likely than not does little more than increase a level of misery that is already too painful.

2. Frustration and aggression. To keep from rewarding aggression is one thing; to deal with deep and long-lasting frustrations that drive people to aggression is another. Aggression is a very likely response to frustration; the stronger the strength of the frustrated drive and the longer the period of frustration, the more likely the aggression. These are propositions fully elaborated by

Dollard and his associates (1938) many years ago. Subsequent research, not to mention the events of the day, have strongly confirmed them. It has been pointed out that the more arbitrary the frustration, the more likely the aggression—a point well illustrated in some urban riot behavior. The most miserable and totally crushed ghetto residents are less likely to riot than are those who have climbed a rung or two up the ladder, only to find that further progress is blocked. Their aroused expectations make further frustration seem very arbitrary indeed.

To understand violence in city life today, one has to see the interacting influences of the two forms of aggression we have thus far described. Frustration-induced aggression is the basic problem, and can be eliminated only as the larger society eliminates the misery of the ghetto. The force of that aggression and its frequency depend on whether or not ghetto residents discover that their only instrument for effecting change is violence. An additional complexity is the effect of punishment. Oddly enough, city fathers can both reward and punish the same violent demonstrations, fulfilling demands that are made and punishing individual rioters. Since punishment increases frustration and reward reinforces behavior, the effect is to double the likelihood of future aggression.

No one should assume that a simple explanation of the dynamics of the problem will solve it. But neither should we underestimate the value of such understanding in leading us to the difficult solution we must find, particularly when some people (even political leaders) seem to think that a few civil-rights acts have decreased all causes of complaint and frustration.

3. Aggression as a function of obedience. Complexity is compounded by Milgram's finding that obedience to strong social expectations can produce aggression. In ingenious and elaborately designed experiments, Milgram (1963, 1965) was able to show that a group of average Americans, feeling no strong anger or frustration, committed what they believed were extreme acts of aggression against innocent peers. The motivation for the behavior was the demands of the role they had accepted, backed by social pressures, with overtones of prestige, institutional support, and socially valuable goals. The subjects were told by a scientist of Yale University to administer extreme and possibly dangerous electric shocks to another person in order to complete a scientific study on learning. Almost two-thirds of the group complied. Even in later studies, when the institutional props of the university were removed and the studies were done in low-prestige surroundings, aggression in response to obedience occurred.

Outside the laboratory situation, there are comparable pressures on people to be aggressive. The roles of policeman, soldier, union leader, or community leader may be perceived as demanding aggressive behavior. The more the society, through mass media of communication, portrays those roles in aggressive activities, the greater is the pressure of people in the roles to be aggressive.

Obedience to perceived role demands, supported by awareness of other forms of socially approved aggression, feeds into the other two factors we have described to exacerbate urban problems of hate and violence. The implications for social action seem clear to us.

4. Aggression as a function of imitation (social learning). Aggressive responses may occur because one has seen these responses made by someone else. If a variety of possible responses or mechanisms is available, the probability that aggressive behavior will be chosen is increased when violence has been observed either directly or portrayed through the mass media.[6]

One illustrative study (Bandura et al., 1961) had children observe a model behaving in novel aggressive ways that had previously had very low probabilities of occurrence. The same sorts of aggressive verbal and motor responses were quite clearly induced in the children. In addition, compared to control and to nonaggressive model groups, approximately twice as much general aggression was shown by the children who had an aggressive model to imitate. Thus, social learning or imitation, as well as instrumental learning, can increase aggression. The effects of imitation, or modeling, of aggressive behavior cannot be ignored, whether one considers aggression instrumental behavior that is rewarded perhaps by social approval, as obedience to what seem to be the prevailing norms or to the role demands, or as response to frustration.

There has been much argument about the influence of the mass media in producing aggressive behavior. Some have held that there is a cathartic effect in the vicarious release of the viewers' pentup hostility; others argue that the chief effect is imitation.

[6]The relevant research of Bandura and his associates on imitation, and of Berkowitz and others on aggression, is effectively surveyed by Sechrest and Wallace (1967) and by Tannenbaum and Greenberg (1968).

Tannenbaum and Greenberg (1968) indicate that there is considerable research that should lead to rejecting the catharsis effect; they strongly suggest the opposite influence: that observed violence predisposes toward more aggressive behavior. In their view:

Whatever their shortcomings the data in hand are more impressive than mere anecdote and speculation. In particular, the several justification experiments point to the paradox that, in their depictions of "Crime doesn't pay," the media may actually be undermining the very moral and behavioral qualities they seek to promote (Tannenbaum and Greenberg, 1968, p. 351).

The Berkowitz studies are cited to show that "cloaking the violence in a mantle of acceptability" promotes more aggressive behavior on the part of the viewer.

Elsewhere, Watson has pointed out that:

the average American child, watching the most popular television program for the average period of time during his formative years will probably witness the destruction of some 13,000 individuals. This probably exceeds, quantitatively the exposure to scenes of violence experienced by the youth of any other society of which we have records (Watson, 1966, p. 295).

To which we might add: Could that many scenes of reconciliation of differences by peaceful means be seen? We doubt it.

All behavior observed does not lead to imitated behavior. As Sechrest and Wallace (1967, p. 143) point out, the consequences for the model are an important consideration. Of relevance here is Wertham's (1962) point that television often shows the violence without showing its bloody, painful, harmful, or long-lasting consequences. The violence is seen as amusing or justified, not as damaging to a human being.

Another determinant of whether behavior will or will not be imitated is who the model is. The model with prestige or in control of rewarding reinforcement is more readily imitated than the model who is not (Sechrest & Wallace, 1967, p. 143). One question not answered is whether appearance per se in any medium gives prestige for some to an aggression model.

In general, it seems safe to hypothesize that the more socially approved forms of aggression a society tolerates in any area, and the more examples of aggression shown to its members (in any medium), the more aggressive behavior will spread into all other social activities. Ghetto teenagers viewing war activities find it easier to throw bricks.

5. *The aggressive personality.* Aggressive sociopaths contribute to the hate-violence syndrome because of leadership roles they can assume. Psychiatrists have identified a group of people whose first impulsive response to any sort of blocking is aggression. In general, they have little ego-strength, no capacity to delay gratification of their needs, and little ability to discriminate between one situation and another. Their world is cast in deep contrasts—good and bad, yours and mine, the in-group and the out-group. Their regular response to any tension is aggression. When they respond as individuals, the problem is a psychiatric one, frequently involving police action and criminal charges. When their own aggressions affect the behavior of groups in which they hold influential positions, the problem is different and more serious. We want to be very careful here to state that urban groups are no more subject to influence by sociopathic personalities than are any other groups in our society. Nevertheless, in any listing of factors leading to hate and violence, the effect of emotional illness must be noted.

An Experimental Approach: Testing the Effectiveness of Different Approaches to an Urban Problem

Practically any administrative decision aimed at dealing with a specific problem has an implicit (or explicit) theory about behavior as its basis. Our theme throughout the chapter has been the use of behavioral-science data as an important basis for urban decisions. Here we take a specific problem for illustrative purposes, and outline an experimental test of ways of dealing with that problem. Whether our design or the techniques tested are the best is secondary to our purpose of encouraging the view that urban problems are amenable to and appropriate for research. Our description assumes that a search of the literature for earlier related behavioral work has already been done.

A dangerous and costly form of behavior in cities is the turning in of false fire alarms. The false-alarm rate can, if one chooses, be viewed as a symptom of community mental health. Assuming that one is dealing with a city that has relatively clear-cut and separate districts, it is possible to try out different approaches to reducing false alarms in different matched areas, and to use changes in the false-alarm rate as criteria for assessing the relative effectiveness of the various approaches. The experiment would begin with careful selection of specific approaches to be tested. Some approaches obviously "treat the symptom" directly; others aim at some of the presumed underlying problems. In either case, expert opinion and prior experience, if any, would suggest which approaches are most promising.

For illustrative purposes, we suggest five approaches to the false-alarm problem that might be evaluated, and also suggest the psychological premise in developing each approach.

1. The noise-making approach. It is possible to design fire-alarm boxes so that not only does the firehouse get a report but the box itself emits some loud noise, such as a bell ringing or a siren. The apparently obvious behavioral-science premise here is that to avoid the negative reinforcement of being caught (presumably made more likely by the immediate noise produced), possible offenders are deterred.

As is sometimes the case, another, and contradictory, set of premises might be suggested as applicable, with quite different results. If one assumes that some alarms are turned in by those seeking "kicks" (not necessarily adolescents) or by those seeking attention (perhaps from peers who are watching), then the noise is positive, not negative reinforcement. The false-alarm rate might drop if negative reinforcement is anticipated, or rise if positive reinforcement is experienced.

The possibility of both effects—that is, noise serving to deter some people and reward others—might even mean no rate change, with no easy way of disentangling the differential influence of the technique to see what future modifications might accomplish (and no significant effect on the problem, in any immediate sense).

2. The community-recreation approach. Another technique would be to "saturate" a community with a variety of recreational facilities. The underlying concepts here are recognizable as frustration reduction, as well as the provision of substitute activities. Other premises, related to the age and other features of offenders, are involved, and could lead to testing the effectiveness of special facilities for children, teenagers, older people, alcoholics, addicts, and so on. The technique is obviously indirect, not symptom-oriented, long-range in its effect, and costly.

3. Attitude studies. Attitude surveys represent another approach, the attempt to determine the attitudes of firemen toward the people in the community and, in turn, the attitudes of the community toward firemen (see Bard, 1967). This technique assumes that follow-up programs would be developed based on survey findings (for example, role playing; sensitivity training; community activity). From a conceptual viewpoint, the approach assumes that the behavior and attitudes of firemen in the community influence the people in the area, and that improved understanding of the neighborhood by firemen would reduce such hostile acts as false alarms.

4. Use of the firehouse for other community purposes. In this approach, amusement, education, or assistance for the community might be promoted in the firehouse. For example, little-used areas in the firehouse might be used for dances, movies, shows, or other entertainment. Locally helpful information, special open meetings or courses on schooling, training, how to get jobs, how to fill out tax forms, hobbies, home repairs would be available at the firehouse. It is apparent here that the attempt is to increase friendly interaction between the neighborhood people and the firemen through a community-center approach. Theoretical bases include not only frustration reduction, but the development of trust and friendship within both the community and the fire department, as well as the association of the fire department with pleasant or helpful activities.

5. Local publicity campaigns. Both traditional and innovative local publicity campaigns on the hazards, costs, and problems of false alarms represent another approach. The local, rather than the widespread, campaign is suggested to reduce experimental-design problems. Publicity could be varied, among other ways, in media used (printed, sound-truck), location (house-to-house, at fire-alarm boxes), style ("scare" or mild tone content, the latter emphasizing cost and helping families), degree of local participation (leaflets handed out by firemen, teenagers, firemen's children).

Let us sketch in some of the controls that would be required in a comparative test of the five approaches suggested. It would be necessary to try out each approach in a separate area of the city (preferably not a separate city, to prevent the introduction of other variables), to seek to avoid any publicity about the experiment, and to set up procedures to reduce the likelihood of communication from one area to another about the study within the fire department. It would be important for those cooperating in different areas not to inform people in the communities of the study.

Since the introduction of *any* plan can have consequences (a Hawthorne effect), it would be necessary (1) to have a control-group area or district where no change is being made, and (2) to keep the community and firemen from knowing that they are part of an experiment on false alarms (except for the publicity approach, where awareness is inevitable). For some of the approaches, unawareness of the purpose is easy to ensure. In providing recreational facilities, for example, there certainly need be no mention of fire alarms.

In a more idealized but less feasible form, one would like to see groups who thought they were part of an experiment: one with nothing changed; a second where they were given a "positive" set on the potential of the experiment; and a third where a "negative" set was given ("We don't think it will work, but let's try it."). Other niceties of experimental design are unlikely to be possible in a field experiment.

The major criterion of the relative effectiveness of the various approaches would be the *changes* in the false-alarm rates. This in part helps to avoid such problems as setting up matching districts with comparable original rates, comparable types or accessibility of alarm boxes; and comparable age, income, or ethnic groupings in the areas.

The false-alarm rate is a convenient dependent variable that can be used in many cities without alerting anyone to the fact that an experiment is under way, since the data are gathered routinely and can be obtained long after the introduction of the experimental approaches, without a change in municipal procedures. In some cities, there are data on the specific boxes with the largest false-alarm rates; such data are particularly useful.

Some secondary or additional criteria would be relevant: vandalism, specifically against fire-department property; attacks on firemen; change in the number of real fires not reported, or reported only after extensive damage; change in the number of false alarms received in other ways, as by telephone calls.

One perennial measurement problem concerns when to take criterion measures. Some experimental approaches might show initial or early declines in the rate of false alarms, and then later increments. Others might be slow in producing any change. What is called for would be more than a "one-shot" time-interval choice, with different seasons of the year represented, for instance.

In a field study, it is obviously necessary to keep track of any other community changes and influences that might affect the criterion besides the experimental approaches (and to hope that the "outside influences" would either be minimal or similar for all areas of the experiment). Anyone planning a field experiment of the sort we have outlined would naturally be faced with the usual variety of dilemmas and decisions. We have by no means sought to fill in all details or indicate all the relevant variables. In choosing the fire-alarm problem, we do not necessarily believe our example identifies the most fruitful beginning for true experimental work on urban problems. We use it to argue a simple case.

The usual approaches taken to urban problems have a certain logic to them. Decisions are made that take assumptions as fact. Experience in many other areas suggests that, often, fact can only be verified through experimental testing. We believe that community mental-health workers can effectively develop some of those experimental approaches as part of their community work.

CONCLUSION

We have tried in this chapter to weave together three significant strands of modern life: the urban crisis, behavioral-science research, and community mental-health practice. We have blocked out some ways of thinking about cities and some conditions that handicap problem-solving efforts. Legislative and fiscal solutions are needed, but behavioral science can make important contributions. We have examined a variety of these, and illustrated two research approaches in more detail.

In all of this the community mental-health worker plays a significant part. His practice is more likely than not to be in an urban setting. Problems faced by cities handicap his efforts. Progress made in behavioral science can enhance them. The community mental-health field—because it interfaces with both municipal government and behavioral science—can provide the bridge between the two.

REFERENCES

Bandura, A., Ross, S., & Ross, S. Transmission of aggression through imitation of aggressive models. *J. abnorm. soc. Psychol.,* 1961, **63**, 575-582.

Bard, M. Training police as specialists in family crisis intervention: community psychology action program. *Community ment. Hlth J.,* 1967, 3 (4), 315-317.

Berelson, B., & Steiner, G. *Human behavior—an inventory of scientific facts.* New York: Harcourt, Brace & World, 1964.

Berkowitz, L. *Aggression: a social psychological analysis.* New York: McGraw-Hill, 1962.

Blank, Blanche. Personal communication, 1966.

Catton, B. *A stillness at Appomattox.* New York: Doubleday, 1953.

Costello, T. W., & Zalkind, S. S. *Psychology in administration—a research orientation.* Englewood Cliffs, N.J.: Prentice-Hall, 1963.

Costello, T. W., & Zalkind, S. S. Urban problems and behavioral science research. *Management Sci.,* 1968, **14** (8), 8415-8422.

Dollard, J., Doob, L. W., Miller, N. E., Mowrer, O. H., & Sears, R. R. *Frustration and aggression.* New Haven: Yale Univer. Press, 1938.

Gruen, V. *The heart of our cities—the urban crisis: diagnosis and cure.* New York: Simon & Schuster, 1964.

Hilgard, E. R., & Atkinson, R. C. *Introduction to psychology.* (4th ed.) New York: Harcourt, Brace & World, 1967.

Hollingshead, A. B., & Redlich, F. C. *Social class and mental illness.* New York: Wiley, 1958.

Katz, D. The functional approach to the study of attitudes. *Publ. Opin. Quart.,* 1960, **24**, 163-204. Reprinted in T. W. Costello & S. S. Zalkind, *Psychology in administration—a research orientation.* Englewood Cliffs, N.J.: Prentice-Hall, 1963, pp. 250-260, 265-274.

Lazarsfeld, P.F. Sociological reflections on business. In R. A. Dahl, M. Haire, & P. F. Lazarsfeld, *Social science research on business: product and potential.* New York: Columbia Univer. Press, 1959. Pp. 99-153.

McNeil, E. B. Psychological aggression. *J. of Conflict Resolution,* 1959, **3**, 195-293. Abridged in T. W. Costello & S. S. Zalkind, *Psychology in administration—a research orientation.* Englewood Cliffs, N.J.: Prentice-Hall, 1963, pp. 139-147.

Milgram, S. Behavioral study of obedience. *J. abnorm. soc. Psychol.,* 1963, **67**, 371-378.

Milgram, S. Some conditions of obedience and disobedience to authority. *Human Relat.,* 1965, **18**, 57-76.

Montagu, M. F. A. (Ed.) *Man and aggression.* New York: Oxford Univer. Press, 1968.

Moynihan, D. P. New racialism. *Atlantic,* 1958, **222**, 35-40.

Riecken, H. W. Survey of the behavioral and social sciences. *Items* (Soc. Sci. Res. Council), 1966, **20** (4), 45-54.

Russell, B. *Power.* New York: Barnes & Noble, 1962.

Scott, J. P. *Aggression.* Chicago: Univer. of Chicago Press, 1958.

Sechrest, L., & Wallace, J. *Psychology and human problems.* Columbus: Charles E. Merrill Books, 1967.

Tannenbaum, P. H., & Greenberg, B. S. Mass communication. *Annu. Rev. Psychol.,* 1968, 19, 351-386.

Watson, G. *Social psychology.* Phila.: Lippincott, 1966.

Wertham, F. The scientific study of mass media effects. *Amer. J. Psychiat.,* 1962, 119, 306-311; as cited in P. H. Tannenbaum & B. S. Greenberg, Mass communication. *Annu. Rev. Psychol.,* 1968, 19, 351-386, at p. 373.

Wolman, A., Metabolism of cities. *Scientific American,* 1965, 213, 178-188.

CHAPTER 11

The Multiproblem
Neighborhood Project

William C. Rhodes, Julius Seeman, Charles D.
Spielberger, and Robert F. Stepbach, Jr.

This paper is a conceptual analysis of a research demonstration project which explored and attempted to influence the human-trouble handling machinery of a community. The project, which focused upon a multiproblem neighborhood, served as the behavioral science resources of the university and the human-disruption control machinery of the community. However, in addition to its transmission function, the project had a significant generative function in both of these separate systems. The project pivoted around a demographic data-gathering effort which was an important aspect of its existence. This data will be published separately in a later report; our purpose here is to set forth a conceptual model which has generality beyond the project itself.

CONCEPTUAL OVERVIEW

A Macrosystem Model

The project was based upon the concept that community agencies and human-service programs function not only to help people in trouble but also to protect the community against the perceived threats of problem-producers. The agitated encounters between stress excitors and strain-respondent segments of the community were our subject matter in a macrosystem that involved a number of different components:

Reprinted with permission of the authors and Behavioral Publications, from *Community Mental Health Journal*, Vol. 4, No. 1 (February 1968), pp. 3-12.

1. Enclaves of psychocultural stressors or threat-elicitors in the larger community; that is, the multiproblem neighborhoods;

2. A community interlace of specialized threat-respondent units (the community agencies) that act in concert with;

3. The power structures of the community (governmental and specialized human-service agencies) in behalf of the general public who constitute the strain-respondent groups of the community.

This self-maintaining macrosystem of community threat and response may be construed as resulting from the gradual institutionalizing or hardening of a widening cleavage between the life history of individuals and the cultural history of the community. In order to clarify the elements of this conceptual model and the linkages among them, it is necessary to offer a brief description of each of the three units.

The multiproblem neighborhood. This consists of area clusters of threat-elicitors who are inadequate, emotionally disturbed, economically deprived, or who have frequent physical health emergencies or difficulty with the law, etc. The major groups of the community respond to personal-social disruptions in these areas as though a strain was being placed upon the collective community. Thus, the threat elicitors constitute a catabolic force in community living that heightens cleavages within the community.

The culturing institutions. In this particular model of ecological disruption-response, the disruption-handling elements of the culturing institutions constitute the defense machinery which is erected against a perceived danger. Operational patterns of social welfare, legal-correction, mental health, public health, education, housing, recreation, and religion all contribute their share to this defensive array. Varying portions of the resources and culturing forces of these social institutions are devoted to the defensive task.

The power structures. All of the defensive patterns of the community interlock with the power structures of the community to prevent major disjunctions between the individual and collective living. Some of the personal-social disruptions to which this machinery responds, such as mob violence, may constitute real dangers to group living. Others, such as homosexuality, may be remnants of a past historical period. For the latter, the actual threat may not justify the institutional response.

Linkages in the Disruption-Handling Machinery

Since the executive direction of the trouble-handling or disruption-control machinery is rarely located at the neighborhood level, the mobilization and deployment of the neighborhood forces are directed from an echelon outside the neighborhood context. The decision-making apparatus of the disruption-handling machinery is generally made up of agency executives and their boards. The agency executives are linked to the community power structure through liaison with the executive, judicial, and legislative branches of government. They relate to the informal power structures of the community through their own policy-making boards.

In collaboration with the formal and informal power structures, the disruption-handling machinery of the community defends against collectively real and fantasied threats from the disruption-producing neighborhoods. These power structures are the seat of the major decisions about when, how, where, and how much of the community's resources will be mobilized and deployed in front-line defense against particular threats at the neighborhood level. While there is some autonomy at each level of the defensive machinery, much of the strategy is determined and directed from the upper echelons, particularly at the level of executive, legislative, and judicial governmental organization. These determinations usually are consolidated into laws which form the basis for community relationships with the disrupting populations.

In order to enter this total human control system and insure its cooperation at the neighborhood level, it is generally necessary to obtain the sanction of the upper agency echelon as well as the relevant, formal, and informal power structure levels. Whatever is done at the neighborhood level is quickly communicated up the communication lines of the system, and if an action is perceived as inimical to the directions and decisions of the upper echelons, it is likely to invoke resistance and rejection.

Therefore, unless one is prepared to meet and overcome such resistance, or to work outside the human disruption system and its sanctions, it is necessary to achieve and maintain the approval of the community power structure for one's operations.

Guided by this macrosystem model, the project not only concentrated upon a particular multiproblem neighborhood but also devoted considerable time and negotiation at two other crucial entry points into the system of disruption control, namely, the executive branch of local government and the executive units of the major disruption control or threat-respondent units such as police, welfare, education, health, etc. This was seen as a necessary part of the project and influenced both staffing and organization of the project structure.

The Problem Unit

The major conceptual difficulty was, from the very beginning of the project, the nature of the disruptions which were the focus of concern. The pivotal concept with which the project began was that of "discordance." Initially the phenomenon which was to have our major attention was described as "discordant behavior." This term was used to bracket a number of psychosocial problems which seemed related to each other and to the debilitating conditions of a "slum" habitat. Discordant behavior included delinquency, alcoholism, psychosis, crime, desertion, etc., as well as any other behaviors and patterns of living that were discordant with the standards of the community.

We recognized, of course, that the concept of discordance implies culturally relative terms. "Delinquency," for example, might be defined differently in two different communities, according to the local legal code. To meet the problem of relativeness, we used the term "discordant behavior" to refer to specific episodes or incidents. These episodes were defined in terms of a traumatic human event which elicited a response from one or more of the community agencies established by society to deal with that class of upsetting human events.

Thus, for our purpose, the response by an appointed agent of the community was the operational definer of an event as discordant with community behavioral standards.

Two problems were encountered in the use of the discordance concept. One problem was that some of the human events which aroused agency response did not conform to the discordance concept in that they did not violate community norms, taboos, or sanctions. Many simple life episodes, such as a loss of a pair of glasses by an elderly resident of the community, were judged as significant disruptions by the official agent; whereas, in the beginning, it seemed almost irrelevant to the study group.

A second problem concerned the relativity of the discordance concept. It was surprising how perspective and base lines shifted once the study group became immersed in the culture of the neighborhood. What seemed dissonant or discordant prior to such immersion became a normal way of life or a normal part of life after immersion.

After the pilot data were collected, studied, and analyzed, it became evident that the episodes, which had been collected through the wide net of the total gamut of neighborhood based community agents, were stretching the limits of the working concept. Discordance, as the major concept, did not capture the full range of the data. The life happenings within the neighborhood which activated agencies or which demanded community response were definitely within the realm of personal-social disruptions, but they were of a wider ecological nature. While they all had psychosocial repercussions, not all of them were psychosocial in essence.

An arbitrary choice could have been made to include only episodes of a psychosocial nature, but then much rich and significant data would have to be ignored. Furthermore, these psychosocial disruptions were entwined within a nest of disruptions, so that it was very hard to separate them out as a pure case of the class we wanted. Even more important, an episode frequently had a fluidity that would not permit the time-demarcation of a beginning and end which would separate off the psychosocial from the physical, the economic, the legal, etc. Like a chameleon, an episode frequently reflected different colors from moment to moment or even at the same moment "in situ," so that it was hard to pin it down into an unchanging class. It became important, therefore, to shift to an ecological frame of reference and to a concept of a normal, but fluid, individual and group functioning within the neighborhood and family milieu.

Therefore, at the point of the collection of the first-run data, the concept of *Ecological Disruption* seemed to be more useful. "Ecological" signified the relationship between the individual and his environment and between persons and community. An ecological disruption was defined as any human-centered event that interrupted the relative steady state of the neighborhood to such an extent that it elicited a response from a local caretaker. Thus, each recorded event had two sets of terms—the excitor terms and the respondent terms, and each recording of an ecological disruption specified properties of both the excitor and the respondent.

PROJECT OVERVIEW

The Neighborhood Site Focus

Before going further into a description of the project, the authors acknowledge the limitations of their approach. It is recognized that to look at the process of individual disruptions and community response is merely to view the existing practices and problem-conceptions of communities. It does not uncover more significant or neglected human problems in these zones of problem concentration. However, this approach did engage the macrosystem of disruption handling, while avoiding collision or conflict with the system, and it allowed us to move inside the system and observe and record its operations first hand.

The geographical unit chosen as the site for recording and mapping these excitor-respondent episodes was a multiproblem or high-disruption producing neighborhood with a high concentration of disruption-handling machinery. The machinery consisted of police, social welfare, housing, health, and other agencies. The area was one of the three trouble-producing neighborhoods in the community in a moderate size metropolitan area of 460,000 population. It was selected on the basis of the following criteria: (*a*) contain a high density of indigenous multiproblem behavior; (*b*) manifest high community agency involvement; (*c*) be predominately a single race neighborhood; (*d*) contain a public low-rent housing project; (*e*) contain a community center; (*f*) be accessible to the university, and limited in areas so that it can be covered on foot.

The first two criteria comprise the major components of the study and are obviously required. Criterion *c* was included to limit the number of variables to be studied. Criterion *d* was included because it had been observed that multiproblem families and associated agency involvement are concentrated in public housing projects. Criterion *e* was included because of its strategic value as a base of observation. The final criterion was directed toward the question of accessibility and efficiency of staff utilization.

The Project Apparatus

The project brought together the university resources on one hand and representatives of the disruption-handling machinery of the community on the other. On the university side there was an advisory group and a project director. Represented in the university segments were:

1. The sociology and psychology departments of one institution.
2. The psychology department of a second institution.
3. The department of psychiatry at a third.
4. Staff members of the community's mental health center.

On the community side, the involvement included:

1. The congeries of neighborhood based operations of the human-service agencies (representing the "caretaker" group).
2. The executives and their boards in the official disruption-handling machinery of human-service agencies. (The middle-management group.)
3. That part of the official community power structure devoted to the handling of disruptions between individuals and community.

The representatives of the university had several functional connections with various levels of the community disruption-handling machinery. University faculty were on various committees of the governing body of the city, and on various committees established for the regular functioning of the middle-management group in executive control of the agencies. In addition, each of the executives of the agencies with official responsibility for disruption-control were formally contacted and involved in the project. Some of these executives served for varying periods of time and for specific purposes on the Directorate Group of the project. The agencies included health, mental health, education, welfare, housing, etc.

Neighborhood Level Procedures

At the neighborhood level, a full-time and a half-time participant-observer were the mainsprings of the project throughout the full year. The full-time neighborhood participant-observer was an advanced student with training in psychology and sociology. The half-time participant-observer was an experienced degree psychologist on the staff of the local mental health center with responsibilities as a clinician and a community consultant. He was well known in the community and had a wide range of established relationships with all levels of the disruption-handling machinery.

The two key project staff members functioned in the neighborhood in a semiautonomous role. That is, they were identified as project personnel associated with a study conducted from the university center, and they also established loose ties to the caretaker group in the neighborhood. Their major identifiable relationship unit was a Neighborhood Council of the caretaker group.

Considerable time was spent in the initial stages of the project just "hanging around" in the neighborhood. The two participant-observers also moved around the neighborhood streets, hang-outs, and institutional centers. They became familiar with the ministers, police, housing authorities, health workers, case workers, barbers, tavern-keepers, etc. In addition to their movable office, they also had space in the local community center (settlement house).

Once the top agency directors of the "middle-management" group had sanctioned the project, each of the caretakers in the neighborhood was contacted on an individual basis. In addition, the project was explained and discussed with the Neighborhood Council.

The major means of initial data collection was a routine intelligence-gathering route traveled daily and/or weekly by one of the participant-observers. In the later research phases, this method was abandoned for a more rigorous and controlled procedure. The senior participant-observer found himself drawn into frequent consultation to the caretaker groups in the neighborhood. Although this was not a planned part of the project, it had been anticipated and was acknowledged to be a necessary reciprocity for the time and interest given the project by the caretaker group. Both the data gathering and the consultation provided a continuing, reciprocal, mutually advantageous relationship between the project and the caretaker group.

A Human Culturing Concordat

Through the two linkage agents, the resources of the university's complex and the resources of the total community disruption-control apparatus were provided with a temporary coupling system. Through this coupling system and this operational focus upon a commonly shared problem, a back-and-forth flow between the two entities was established.

Some of the operational patterns created out of this interchange are discussed below. For the present, however, reflection upon this process suggests that the only additional ingredients needed to consolidate these task-focused alliances into a joint operational organization of some endurance would be: (*a*) a stated agreement between the working parties and (*b*) continuity in funding sources. These ingredients can translate the task-focused cooperative endeavor into almost any desired form of intermediate agency between the university and community machinery, so long as it does not violate the established investments of either party to the agreement.

If our observations are valid, this suggests that it would be possible to establish a blending station or operational center which could channel and provide the appropriate interflow between the human science resources of the university and the disruption-control resources of the community toward specified human culturing ends. Such a center could act as an intermediate switching station between the conceptual and problem-solving skills of the university and the caretaking attitude and functions of the disruption-control machinery. At the same time it could offer a community observatory or laboratory for research and training programs of the university.

In our particular project, the joint endeavor of data-gathering and the two linkage agents accomplished this type of exchange and institute pattern. On one side was the Project Directorate which utilized university faculty from three institutions and four human science departments, and on the other side was the Caretaker Council of the neighborhood and the loose working relationships that were developed with agency executive and the mayor's office. As indicated earlier in this report, although the project focused its efforts upon the neighborhood site, it also devoted considerable time throughout the project period to the other two levels of executive structures mentioned above. We continued to take the position that the disruption-handling network formed a total community Gestalt which was administratively connected in ways not obvious to the outside researcher, and that a research-focused entry point into this network was likely to be felt and known (and possibly resented) by the other parts of the total machinery.

The experience of this temporary coordinate coupler between the university and the disruption control machinery provides suggestions for the multiple ways in which such an interlocutor mechanism might become a generator of evolution and change in the culturing media of communities. Some of the generative effects produced by this project included the following:

1. Sparked a special neighborhood problem-solving subgroup or change-agent committee of the Neighborhood Council of caretakers.

2. Provided the nucleus of a branch unit of the mental health clinic especially designed to reach out into the poverty area and the target population of the poor.

3. Implanted the embryo of a University Center for Community Studies.

4. Provided a psychosocial laboratory in a slum area within which advanced graduate students could obtain supervised Community Psychology experience.

These ripple effects of the project are its most tangible community results. They evolved out of the research-focused exchanges of the university and community groups and are having generative effects of their own upon both the excitor or stress-inducing populations and the disruption-handling machinery of the community. They are also having feedback effects upon the university center.

In order to provide a better grasp of each of these direct organizational outcomes of the project, a brief description of each is given below.

The Neighborhood Change Agent Committee

The "Change Agent Committee" of the Neighborhood Council arose out of the revitalized interest of the Council members in neighborhood planning. A small number of members formed a subgroup of the Council and agreed to meet weekly for lunch and discussion. The Committee has been and is presently composed of the following types of caretakers: a public housing project manager, the director of a neighborhood settlement house, a housing project social service worker, a public welfare worker, a psychiatric social worker, and a clinical/community psychologist. Additional professional people have met with the group from time to time to help the Committee clarify issues in which there was a lack of competency. An example of one such meeting was a lengthy discussion with an attorney during which time he expertly discussed in lay terms the social dilemmas of legal aid, divorces for the poor, garnishment, bankruptcy, loan practices, usury, and more.

Currently, the Committee has proposed a twofold plan for neighborhood action. First, they intend to emphasize the development of self-governing and self-determining groups. People with problems will be the problem solvers whenever possible. Experts will be used to facilitate this process as necessary. Increased socialization and the restoration of self-dignity and purpose are the obvious goal of this part of the plan.

Secondly, increased communication among agencies serving the neighborhood has been planned. A workable, neighborhood central clearing house for problem families has been proposed out of which coordinated service and planning can emanate. In addition, a serious effort will be made to ask and provide answers to "researchable" questions. For example, by studying gaps in agency services and families who fall through the "cracks," it is hoped that meaningful data will be provided the policy-making bodies of the community. They, in turn, can generate sound legislation which will enhance the welfare of the neighborhood.

It is apparent that the Neighborhood Council has become more than a monthly meeting of caretakers offering mutual emotional support in the face of overwhelming professional problems. It has become a springboard for social action, a kind of middleman between the clients and the agency policy makers who spell out the types of services offered to those clients.

Branch Neighborhood Counseling Center

The branch unit of the Mental Health Center is calling itself a Neighborhood Counseling Center in order to minimize the fear and avoidance people feel about mental and emotional problems. The staff consists of a resident (Negro) psychiatrist from a local medical school, a clinical psychologist, two psychology interns, three psychiatric social workers, and two second year students in social work. The unit is housed in the Manager's Office of the local public housing project. It operates on a half-time basis.

The branch clinic has the task of finding out why the lower class does not use the traditional mental health services in the community. At this stage, a large portion of time is spent in consultation with neighborhood caretakers and community planning. Therapeutic endeavors are experimental, flexible, and adapted to the needs of the person or persons in trouble. An attempt has been made to make treatment a part of the dynamic social process of the neighborhood rather than an isolated phenomenon in a strange office across town.

The Proposed Center for Community Studies

It became clear that the current time-limited project was only one of many possible prototypes for community-oriented research. The conviction grew among the staff that a more permanent organization was needed to bring a behavioral science capability to bear upon community problems. From this conviction grew the idea of a Center for Community Studies.

The purpose of the Center would be to foster inquiry and experimentation in community behavioral processes. The interest areas of the Center would be broad enough to include those community processes where human effectiveness may be enhanced— for example, delinquency, social disorganization, emotional disturbance, poverty, educational problems, and the like.

The foregoing objective makes it clear that the Center's domain of concern would require a broad interdisciplinary research approach. It is envisioned that the staff and consultant organization initially would include at least the disciplines of sociology, psychology, psychiatry, and anthropology. The principle of the Center's staffing would be that the Center could call upon broad knowledge in the behavioral sciences for the studies.

CHAPTER 12

Adults and Adolescents:
An Experiment in Mutual Education

Leonard Hassol

During some ten years of consultation work in American public schools, I have gained the conviction that many of the ways in which the schools relate to children are in direct conflict with democratic values, and especially with those values most strenuously urged upon school children by their teachers. This conflict can be seen in the system of judicial procedure which assumes total freedom from bias and total accuracy of observation and interpretation on the part of school personnel, but considerable evasiveness and evil intent on the part of students. It pervades essentially arbitrary discipline methods which fail to educate either students or teachers about the basic democratic concept of due process. It is present in the colonial structure of student government which retains administrative veto of all student decisions. The ubiquitous system of passes by which students are required to justify divergence from planned schedules speaks volumes about the lip service given to the idea of basic trust. And often a dual standard of conduct is applied as between teachers and students: one might cite here the group of female high-school teachers who told a faculty meeting convened to consider how miniskirts might best be banned, "We'll enforce whatever rules are made for the kids, but don't expect us to dress like a bunch of old maids."

In such circumstances, children do draw conclusions about the real, as opposed to the merely verbal, place which democratic values have in the thoughts and actions of their elders. Friedenberg's studies of American high schools yield clear evidence of the effects of such perceptions upon young people's value systems:

In this world power counts more than legitimacy; if you don't have power it is naive to think you have rights that must be respected ... High school students experience regulation only as control, not as protection. Translated into the high school idiom ... "if you get caught, it's just your ass." Students do not resent this ... they accept school as the way life is and close their minds against the anxiety of perceiving alternatives (Friedenberg, 1965, pp. 47-48).

None of this comes about as a result of any evil intent on the part of school administrators, who are, after all, faced with the task of coping with the emergence, in astronomical numbers, of a generation of adolescents differing in several important respects from any the family of man has heretofore produced. Today's teenagers have an unprecedented degree of mobility, which makes school merely one of many sources of new experience. They have available, via the mass media, enormous amounts of information and stimulation which previous generations would spend a lifetime in acquiring. Some have, through the affluence of their parents, tasted experiences which many previous generations never achieved. They are the beneficiaries of an unprecedented revolution in educational technology. And finally, they have been intimately exposed during the past fifteen years to a condition of permanent reevaluation of most of the social, religious, ethical, and moral underpinnings of organized society. The result has been a determined readiness and an intellectual capacity to question assumptions and fiats about the way things ought to be.

Educators, parents, and others who deal with youth have been hard-pressed to cope with this differently prepared young person, since to do so adequately requires a fundamental shift in one's assumptions and especially one's feelings about young people. Many adults need to learn how to feel comfortable in the presence of the energy, the instinctual drives, and sometimes the youthful arrogance of the adolescent. The well-tuned response to youthful provocation can convert the usual power confrontation into a constructive learning experience. It is in this matter of continued intelligent functioning in the presence of strong emotion that adults can be effective teachers. But if youth looks at age and sees only a reflection of its own weakness, how can it accept the additional experience which is a principal contribution that age can offer youth? In the absence of such adult capacity, there occurs a reinforcing of traditional assumptions about the proper relationship between the adult and adolescent and a rigidifying of efforts at maintaining control at the moment when such methods are showing diminished utility.

The purpose of this chapter is to describe a summer camping experience with 13- and 14-year-olds that may have something to say about alternative ways of bringing adults and adolescents together in a shared learning experience concerning democratic values.

CAMP LEADER LAB

For some years, the Unitarian Universalist Association of New England has conducted a two-week camping experience with youth aged 13 to 15, under the title "Camp Leader Lab." As the somewhat awkward name implies, one purpose of this two-week camping experience is to provide some training and understanding of the problems involved in assuming leadership when the campers return to their year-round youth-group organizations. In past years the essence of what was attempted amounted to somewhat structured discussions under the control of adult staff, most of whom have a combined ministerial and youth-education background. A great deal of talk about leadership and leadership phenomena was encouraged and took place; but never were any opportunities deliberately sought out to experience what actually happens when some people try to lead and others try to follow. Therefore, it was decided to design a modified residential laboratory using sensitivity training[1] as a tool for experiencing and learning about the factors underlying group behavior and personal involvement in groups. The author was engaged as a general consultant to this project.

A word about the structure of Camp Leader Lab would be helpful at this point in understanding the events about to be described. Administratively, the camp was headed by a dean who was appointed by a committee of the sponsoring UUA. He had a volunteer staff made up of ministers and their wives, all of whom had some experience in youth work, and about half of whom had been at past sessions of Leader Lab. Training sessions in T-group theory and technique were conducted by the author during the spring, and a series of T-group sessions was held on the scene

[1]For a theoretical and methodological explanation of sensitivity training, see Schein and Bennis (1965).

during the several days preceding the opening of camp. In the evening hours, after the campers had retired, the staff met for supervision of the day's T-group experiences with the campers and as an ongoing staff T group, designed to deal with problems and issues which emerged as these adults worked at the unsettling task of facing each other and the young people in new ways.

There were 96 campers attending this two-week session, made up of 42 boys and 54 girls all of whom ranged in age from 13 to 15. They came from middle- and upper-middle-class backgrounds, were members of Unitarian-Universalist groups, and were preponderately white in racial composition. Many of them had participated in the liberal religious youth-organization activities of UUA, and were fairly well informed and vocal about many current issues of social concern such as racial conflict, the Vietnam war, and drug use by high-school and college students.

Nine groups were formed, balanced as much as possible on age and sex lines. These groups met for an hour and a quarter each morning with their adult trainer. Prior to each meeting, the author spoke to the entire camp population for ten or fifteen minutes, drawing upon events which had occurred in the several groups of the previous day and weaving them together into some more general principles concerning the functioning of groups. For example, a discussion about the concept of feedback was illustrated by describing a fairly intense argument in the staff group which came about exclusively because one member had interrupted another member before she had finished talking, had made some assumptions about what she had intended to say, and then had reacted in terms of that assumption. The resolution of this situation, which occurred when the trainer suggested that the person who had been interrupted "feed back" what her feelings had been at this interruption, made a very clear teaching point as to the long-range effects on a group's progress of even this kind of relatively mild injured feeling. In the discussion that followed presentation of this incident, a number of the young people verbalized similar situations where they had been unwilling to correct such wrong assumptions about their intentions because their feelings had been bruised by the original brusk cutting off of what they were saying.

During the first few sessions, the young people voiced both discomfort and some anger about the lack of structure to the meetings. Direct comparisons were made with the school situation and the role of the teacher, followed by many puzzled questions about why the trainer was not behaving in a similar manner. However, once it was made clear that the classroom model was not going to be used here, and once matters having to do with developing issues and frictions within the camp activity and daily community life came into discussion, the demand for structure fell away at least for most of the members.

SOME DIFFERENCES BETWEEN TEENAGE AND ADULT GROUPS

Several differences between these teenage groups and adult groups deserve notice. Perhaps not surprisingly, the degree of sheer motor activity accompanying the group sessions was remarkable. While carrying on highly animated discussions of considerable interest to the members, there would still be a tremendous amount of walking around the room, sprawling into many contorted positions, and, on several occasions, going out through the window of a ground-floor room and moving about outside while continuing to participate actively in the group conversation. Of course, this is exactly what these young people do when they are conversing in their informal groups. Once the trainers realized this and stopped questioning the movement, it ceased to be a problem.

A second difference was the rapid pace, during most sessions, at which topics of conversation changed. To the adult trainers, there often seemed to be no apparent connection between the shifts, and yet the young people moved with them in a way that made it clear that to them the meaning was not really changing. An analogy comes to mind of the situation of an observer watching a flock of pigeons on the grass who abruptly and in unison start to fly, even though the observer had detected no disturbing stimulus. In a like manner, these young people seemed to respond to minimal cues which kept them informed of the underlying meaning even as the surface activities seem to boil over into apparently aimless and rapid changes. After a while, the trainers decided to take the obvious step of asking the group what they were up to when some of these puzzling changes took place, and invariably a reasonable answer was forthcoming. It is hard to know at precisely what age this "imprinted" ability to "swing with the crowd" is blunted, but it must be somewhere between 15 and 25. It also may be that given sufficient exposure to young people of this age range, adults may recover this ability. Alternatively, the postverbal generation may be permanently beyond us.

While the initial response of most of these young people to the T-group situation was one of a greater degree of restraint and indeed mistrust than is usually seen with adult groups, it was also observed that when the early issues of trust in one another and in the T-group situation had been mastered, these adolescents were far more ready than adults usually are to apply what they were learning to the rest of their daily experiences. Once convinced that something of value was in hand, that there was a payoff to what these adults were trying to do with them, the young people were quite ready to open themselves to new experience and new ways of relating to one another. By the end of the first week, a majority of the participants showed significant learning around the T-group situation—so much so, indeed, that the staff was able to make use of the T groups as their primary means of communicating with the campers about many issues of camp life which ordinarily would have been dealt with by more directive and authoritative techniques.

THREE INCIDENTS ILLUSTRATING
T-GROUP EFFECTIVENESS

To illuminate the issue posed above, three incidents, drawn from among many, will be presented in some detail and commented upon from the point of view of alternatives to more or less traditional methods of dealing with questions of self-control and social conscience in adolescence.

Incident #1: Cliques in the Dining Room

Fairly early in the life of the camp, the staff became aware of the fact that small cliques were forming in the dining room and at many other camp activities, in which members of an in-group were reaping maximum participation and pleasure from the camp experiences, while many other campers were suffering silently about exclusion from one or another activity or interpersonal participation. This kind of behavior is, of course, often seen among adolescents. After some discussion within the staff, a strategy was evolved for utilizing the T groups to make a learning situation out of this circumstance for everyone present.

The issue of these in- and out-groups was simply raised by the

T-group trainers in a matter-of-fact way with a question as to why it was happening. Members of the in-group were quick to respond with a variety of statements, of which the following are typical. "It's not that we don't like these other kids; it's just that we know each other; we are the swingers; we know all the 'in' ideas and they don't; we were here last year, so naturally we like each other's company better; we just feel good together and don't need any outsiders." The youngsters in the groups who were not part of the clique looked visibly uncomfortable, but could say very little.

The trainers then responded with all the emotional intensity they could muster in somewhat the following terms. "I've been listening to this stuff for about five minutes, and you know what it sounds like to me? It sounds like just what happens when some nigger tries to move into a lily-white neighborhood." This intervention was intentionally worded in this manner for two good reasons: (1) the reaction of exclusiveness was indeed a sample of prejudiced thinking, and (2) almost all of these youngsters held as a cardinal principle of their own self-image freedom from race prejudice, and indeed freedom from most of what they saw as prejudiced thinking in the adult world. They would probably have preferred to be accused of some major felony rather than of genuinely prejudiced thinking. The response was one of great anger and great denial, with strong efforts at reinforcement of their previous rationalizations. The trainers responded by simply turning to those members of the T group who were not part of the "swingers" and asking them how they felt when they were not permitted to sit at the dining-room tables they chose or to join the activity groups they were interested in. These youngsters were now able to verbalize their feelings of rejection and hurt and to say, as one did—when told "I had no intentions of hurting your feelings"—"Well, whether you intended to or not, that's exactly what you did."

The trainers then invited some of the members of the in-group to recall whether they themselves had ever been kept out and, more importantly, how it felt. Thoughtful agreement was then forthcoming with examples that exclusion did indeed hurt and made the excluded one want to engage in some form of obstruction to group activity. Considerable working and reworking of this issue followed and the trainers had an opportunity to soften their original stand by saying that while they wouldn't accuse the members of being prejudiced, it was indeed a revelation to see how people whose intentions were of the best could still fall victim to a kind of temporary prejudiced attitude. The session at which this all occurred ended, and that very noontime the staff was gratified to see the dissolution of the dining-room cliques and a much more fluid pattern of table occupancy prevail from then to the end of camp. One is tempted to compare the educational benefits of this approach and outcome to what might have been accomplished by a simply issued edict to the effect that there would be no more cliquing at the dining-room table.

Incident #2: Assumed Sexual Deviancy

Our second example illustrates an issue that arises with some frequency in secondary schools and in the adolescent peer group in general; namely, the reactions that are elicited from the teenagers by individual boys and girls who seem, on the basis of surface behavior, to possess characteristics commonly assumed to indicate deviant sexual development, that is, effeminate traits in boys and overly masculine traits in girls. While this is a somewhat hypersensitive issue in American society generally, it is especially so among adolescents who, as a matter of normal developmental-task completion, are working hard to form a stable sexual identification for themselves. As with so many other areas of life, adolescents tend to oversimplify and stereotype this developmental issue in the interest of making their own task less demanding and less anxiety-arousing.

The situation at Camp Leader Lab involved a 15-year-old boy, John, who in most respects looked like a typical, awkward, tall and thin, somewhat pimply youngster in the throes of all the usual physiological changes associated with his age. However, in two respects he was somewhat different; his voice had not yet shown any signs of changing, so that when he spoke, he sounded exactly like a tenor-voiced 8-year-old, and his large-muscle coordination was sufficiently poor that he had almost no aptitude for athletics or dancing, or almost any of the physical activities so ardently engaged in by his peers. It was, however, the high tenor voice and a tendency toward a somewhat fluttering use of his hands when he spoke which led most of the campers to feel uncomfortable in his presence. Their way of handling this discomfort was to make all sorts of allusions to what they perceived as his feminine traits.

Thus it was frequent to hear calls of "Here comes Mrs. Jones" or to see exaggerated body movements and hear imitations of his voice—all of which had the effect of saying that he was a girl rather than a boy. This behavior was rather widespread and came from both sexes with equal frequency. The staff also became aware that there was somewhat more of this kind of behavior coming from those youngsters who were the natural leaders and style-setters within the camp culture. Equally disturbing was John's reaction. He seemed to be falling back on a kind of blanket denial of the reality of the whole experience, in that he would show no response whatsoever to all of this behavior, almost pretending that he didn't hear it or see it. He would continue to appear for all functions, even though he was completely isolated from any significant interaction with the other campers.

In trying to deal with this situation, the staff, in their own T group, had to resolve their own feelings regarding John's situation. It developed that most of them were also uncomfortable with him, and, while controlling their expression of feeling a good deal better than the campers, they were also making the same assumption. After considerable discussion about the pure feeling level, as well as some input on the cognitive side regarding the influence of our puritan and frontier traditions upon cultural expectations of masculinity, several of the staff volunteered to talk with the youngster privately, simply to get a clear picture of what he was really like and to report back to the staff with this information. The essence of their finding was that his interests and desires were similar to most other boys of his age, and the staff finally evolved the hypothesis that the slowness in his voice change was probably the origin of a circular self-fulfilling prophecy situation in which the continued response to the voice in terms of effeminacy gradually began to push the youngster into behavior that looked more and more effeminate.

A strategy was finally evolved which made use of two of the T groups which happened to contain several of the acknowledged teenage leaders and in which John was not a member. In each group the adult trainer raised the question of John's behavior, said that the staff was concerned about his camp experience, and simply asked what the members thought about his situation. After a little difficulty in getting started, all of the interpretations about effeminacy and homosexuality were forthcoming, with much evidence of anxiety and fascination within the group. The trainers were able to draw the group's attention to the signs of discomfort in their own verbal and motor behavior as this topic was discussed, and then to raise the question as to whether or not everybody, when going through the teen years, didn't have occasion to wonder and to be concerned as to whether or not they were "going to make it" as an adequate male or an adequate female and, specifically, whether they would be found acceptable as a sexual partner by the opposite sex.

This led to very intense exploration of past experiences and doubts, with a good deal of support being mobilized within the group for everyone's willingness to reveal some of these inner feelings. The discussion even got around to the whole issue of the wearing of long hair by boys and the blurring of surface distinction in dress and behavior that were currently so popular among the adolescent group and which was visibly evident in many of the members of the group. Some of the girls were able to verbalize the fact that they preferred boys who were not the typical picture of the crewcut football hero. When the emotional climate seemed right, each of the trainers asked the two groups if they would be interested in some factual input from the author concerning sexual development among teenagers. This offer was accepted with frightened delight, and a fifteen-minute presentation was given to each of the T groups concerning the facts of individual differences in secondary sexual maturation, the cultural history of stereotyping concerning what is homosexual and what is heterosexual behavior, and some explanation of the possibility of a person beginning to act the way people indicate to him that they expect him to act by their behavior toward him. The concept of self-definition in terms of perceived social expectations was lightly touched on. Finally, some input was given regarding the bisexual nature of human personality. The T groups then returned to a discussion of what they had heard and to further exploration of their own feelings and past history in this regard. No effort was made to suggest any specific form of action toward John's difficulty.

Once again, the response exceeded the staff's expectations. By the following day, much of the content of the two T groups' discussions had spread through the remainder of the camp, the grapevine indicating that extended discussions went on in the dormitories well into the night and that considerable thinking was going on. A group of the more dominant and athletic boys in camp took John under their wing, proceeded to do such things as giving him lessons in how to shoot a basketball, making sure he was part of their conversational groups on the beach, in the dining hall, and in the dormitories and that he was involved in some of the evening skits and folk-singing activities. Moreover, some of the trend-setting girls were observed during the evening dances to be unobtrusively, but quite definitely, giving John dancing lessons and then making sure that he had an opportunity to dance with a number of the girl campers. Stated in this fashion, the entire thing may seem contrived, but what is difficult to convey is the skill and spontaneity with which the young people did all of this. As far as the staff could determine, there was no prearranged or premeditated discussion about what to do with John. Instead, all of the rehabilitative efforts described came about by an unspoken consensus. The youngsters began to do these things because John's behavior and needs had been brought within the compass of their knowledge about themselves.

Again, it is instructive to compare these procedures with the response to supposed effeminacy in most high schools. The person in question is immediately labeled as a "problem case" and sent to the guidance office or, in more affluent schools, to the psychiatrist or psychologist for "help." His parents are alerted to "potentially serious difficulties with John"; and much snickering conversation develops in the lounges and offices. By this time, John is hopelessly labeled as "queer," and every effort at help only fastens that label a bit tighter. John gets no help (the magician doesn't live who could help him face down such a social reality), and the entire school population loses the chance to discover something about themselves and about their power to help one of their members.

Incident #3: The Question of Teenage Smoking

The third incident relates to the question of the relationship between adolescents and adult authority. This issue was joined around behavior which quite commonly puts teenagers and adults at loggerheads, namely, the question of teenage smoking. A few background facts are necessary. Since all of the buildings at the camp were old frame constructions, a long-standing rule had been in effect prohibiting any smoking in the dormitories or dining room and limiting adult smoking to the outdoor areas and certain selected porches of the main building. Additionally, the literature going to parents describing Camp Leader Lab had stated categorically that smoking by campers would not be permitted. This had been a long-standing rule of the sponsoring association which owned the camp property. About midway through the two-week period, the staff, through a variety of channels, became aware of the fact that there was indeed some smoking going on in the dormitories. The issue was raised by the dean in the camp council, and the young people were willing enough to talk about it with the adults. What emerged was an emotionally intense tangle of conflicting ideas.

Only seven or eight campers were actually involved with the smoking activity, and their identities were known to a good number of the other campers. However, in spite of the readily acknowledged danger to the lives of those in the dormitories, there was tremendous reluctance to enforce a prohibition which almost all of the campers felt was, in most other instances, an irrational extension of adult authority. They had tremendous difficulty in separating their recognition of the danger element from their feelings about the more general adult prohibition against smoking by teenagers. Some of the young people were verbalizing their feelings in terms of the civil-rights protest movement and seeing this issue as a small instance of "holding our protest" against the pressure of the adult world. The dominant theme emerging from these camp-council discussions was one of tremendous ambivalence and conflict; the youngsters could see obvious danger to the community, and yet they could not bring themselves to act against the danger because they saw such action as participating in the enforcement of unnecessary adult authority over teenagers. In an almost pathetically intense manner, one of the boys told the council discussion, "I could never hold my head up again if I gave in on this." With the matter thus deadlocked, the staff held its own discussion to determine where it stood.

There was unanimous staff agreement that the situation could not be left unresolved. There was, for one thing, the very real danger to everyone's life, and there was the specific commitment both to the parents of the campers and to the sponsoring association that smoking would not be permitted. On the other hand, it was recognized that enforcement in any direct sense was probably impossible if the staff had to do the job themselves. Mounting a 24-hour police patrol of the dormitory was impractical, and even if it could be done, this would only set the stage for a battle of wits between the campers and the enforcers—with all the cards clearly in the hands of the campers, at least of those who were engaged in the smoking. The alternatives finally boiled down to either finding some way that would enable the campers to agree to a self-imposed rule against smoking or terminating the camp experience a week early. This latter alternative, obviously of a drastic nature, would have had long-term consequences for future camping sessions. Clearly, the desirable alternative was to find a way to get the young people to resolve their conflictual feelings in favor of the responsible choice. Not only would this be a solution for the immediate issue at hand, but it also could be a valuable long-range learning experience for all of them.

The plan that was developed went somewhat in the following manner. The next day, the issue was specifically raised by the trainers within the sensitivity groups, and the discussion that followed produced all of the questions and all of the conflict that had occurred within the camp-council discussion. The purpose of this procedure was to heighten the tension around the issue and to make it clear to every camper that a real crisis was at hand. No effort was made to push for any solution other than to allow the members to struggle with efforts at planning solutions for themselves. Not one of the nine T groups managed to come to a resolution which they themselves felt to be satisfactory, and thus, by the end of that particular day, everyone in camp was in a high state of disequilibrium concerning what would happen. However, in none of the T groups was the very real possibility that the camp would have to be terminated raised by the trainers. The young people, interestingly enough, never thought of this as a possibility in spite of the fact that all of the situational elements leading to such a conclusion were abundantly clear.

That evening, when all of the campers were assembled in the recreation building, the dean interrupted the dancing and asked for their attention about a matter "of the absolutely highest urgency." It is important to note here that the dean was a person who had a real talent for communicating with young people. There was strong affection as well as respect in their attitude toward him. He proceeded to say to them that he had no solution for the problem that they all faced, but that he felt it was his duty to share with them the full extent of what the staff was going through in trying to come up with an answer. In very direct, emotionally powerful language, he proceeded to describe the efforts of the staff to come to a solution, the real alternatives which existed, and the personal anguish of the staff members over what was happening. He concluded by saying, to an intensely hushed audience, that his purpose was not to force any answers from them, but simply to share with them the full burden that the adults were carrying—"to treat you as much like responsible adults as we possibly can." With that and without asking for any discussion, he left the building and went to where the staff was assembled.

There followed a half-hour of further, very anxious discussion by the staff, with great uncertainty as to what, if anything, was going to happen. Then came a knock on the door, and in came a delegation of about eight campers, both boys and girls, sent officially as representatives of the rest of the camping groups. An intense discussion had taken place among the campers, followed by a vote to the effect that smoking would stop for the remainder of camp. The impact of this scene is hard to describe, except to say that the group of young people were at great pains to tell us what lay behind this decision. With some of the youngsters showing tears in their eyes, they reported that the full disclosure by the dean of how the adult staff was feeling had been extremely moving for all the young people, and that they had no prior realization of what turmoil this issue was stimulating within the adults. It had simply seemed like one more instance of adults trying to get teenagers to "do their dirty work." Another point which had carried great weight was the revelation that the camp might have to be terminated and that when parents and members of the central UUA's staff learned that the rules against smoking had been abridged, there was some real question as to whether there would be any future Camp Leader Labs. It was also clear that the entire group had been reached by the honest statement of the dean concerning the heavy burden of responsibility which the campers' action was placing upon his shoulders. None of them had ever considered that if any person in camp were injured in a fire the responsibility would be directly the dean's; that is, they had not considered this in the context of how it must feel to the person actually faced with this prospect. And, finally, the young people said that this was the first time for most of them that adults had been willing to share their thoughts and their burdens completely with teenagers who were part of that set of responsibilities.

Needless to say, the staff at this point was extremely moved. At one point an offer was made to respond to this camper initiative by relinquishing smoking for the duration of camp by all the staff members. When this effort to respond in a meaningful way to the decision of the young people was reported to the camp council, it was considered and then turned down. One youngster summarized the feeling of the group in private conversation when he said, "Adults don't have to give up all their privileges in order to get along with kids. When I'm an adult, I'm going to expect to be able to do some things that kids can't do. So why should I expect you people to feel any differently?" No specific rules or machinery was set up by the campers to enforce the unanimous decision that there would be no more smoking and, as it turned out, no such machinery was necessary. Smoking as a fulcrum around which struggles between campers and staff could take place simply disappeared.

CONCLUSIONS CONCERNING INTERACTION AND COMMUNICATION

To return to the more general issues which these three incidents were chosen to illustrate, some tentative conclusions can be drawn concerning effective interaction and communication between the generations leading to personal growth and greater self-knowledge for both groups. Underlying all three incidents was a foundation of mutual trust built up within the sensitivity groups. Under conditions of contemporary life, it is rare indeed for children of 14 or 15 and adults of 30 or 40 to experience one another in this way. Those responsible for the administration and organization of our secondary-school systems most especially need to give serious thought to ways and means by which students and their teachers can develop such a sense of mutual trust. Brief experiences such as Camp Leader Lab, even if much more widely available, can only create a readiness on the part of youngsters for such an engagement. Conversely, that readiness can be eroded if during the rest of the year they simply encounter the usual kind of imposed authority.

Deriving from this first point is the interesting idea that youngsters of even 12 or 13 can be included in adult decision making. They are very responsive to having the burdens of adult responsibilities shared with them. When the difficult alternatives and duties facing adults in authority are made clear, these young people are able to respond in a constructive manner. The issue, whatever it might be, is taken out of the context of a win-lose struggle and brought into the context of how both groups can win.

A great deal of effort and time is devoted in secondary schools toward providing assistance for students who are seen as having one form or another of emotional or adjustment problem. Rarely, if at all, is thought given to the possibility of involving that student's peers in the helping process. If, as we have seen, young people can be brought to the point of helping one of their number with a "problem" that is as anxiety-arousing to adolescents as the possibility of homosexuality, then there ought to be a very large area in which less anxiety-arousing, more general kinds of issues can be dealt with in a community context. In addition to assistance for any given individual, everyone else involved learns that he can be of help to others and is exposed to considerable education regarding his own inner sources of anxiety and strength. The person, so assisted, has the invaluable experience of learning that other people in his wider community can be sincerely interested in him and willing to give of themselves in helping him. The preventive implications for mental health and personal effectiveness are obvious, as are the implications for the vast amplification of available helping manpower.

The response of this particular sample of young people to the T-group situation and their ability to take what they learned and make use of it outside the group meeting suggest that the whole area of emotional education is one which needs to be looked into by our school systems. An exclusive focus on subject matter and intellectual content may have already produced an unbalanced kind of education, where large areas of human potentiality are simply overlooked. There is no clear reason why the opportunity to learn about the way people behave in groups, the subtle effects which people have on each other, and to develop skill at communicating one's meaning to others, as well as correctly reading the meaning other people intend to convey, should not be included in standard educational curricula. It may well be true that young people are more open to this kind of education in their early teens than later on in life. This may be the ideal time in which to educate them about the emotional underpinnings of human behavior and to equip them with skills designed to improve their interpersonal competence.

Obviously, no simple transfer can be made from this summer-camp experience to the far more complex social system of the public schools, but several ideas do emerge for consideration by school administrators interested in fostering the commitment of students to the educational enterprise.

Perhaps the most suggestive outcome of the Leader Lab experience concerns the conscious use of adult behavior as an action model for young people. Allowing representatives of the teenage group to participate in staff meetings and to influence staff decisions meant a readiness to expose adult limitations and to share adult decision-making burdens. Such reciprocity in the adult-adolescent relationship produced a powerful impact on the teenagers; once tested and accepted as genuine, it allowed them to think of issues and problems of living in relation to real options and real consequences for themselves rather than merely indulging in the childlike gratifications that come from outwitting or frustrating parent surrogates.

To facilitate such learning requires a willingness by adults to take risks, to engage in what might be termed "creative risk taking," and, therefore, *not* to be in control at all times. Achieving this state of mind is not something that a public-school faculty can come to by mere decision to do so. Clearly, some technique is needed by which students and school personnel can obtain concentrated practice in developing and testing open relationships. And during such a learning period the integrity of the schools' program and community relationships need to be safeguarded. A preliminary device which could meet these needs and also dramatize the commitment to new styles of relationship is the weekend retreat attended by teachers, students, administrators, and school-board members. With the availability of a consultant skilled in helping social systems to explore alternative ways of functioning, a great deal could be done in a relatively short time to start a change process moving.[2] Consider, for example, the variety of interpersonal processes that would emerge as a group of students and teachers struggled with the question of how the traditional grading system might be transformed into a consultation experi-

[2] A major example of such a role is to be found in the Cooperative Project in Educational Development (COPED), a collaborative undertaking of eight universities and some forty public-school systems coordinated by NEA-NTL. *Newsletter of the Conference on Strategies for Educational Change*, Vol. 1, No. 7 & 8, Ohio State University, May and June 1966.

ence where the student learns how to develop and apply criteria for evaluating his own performance—an increasingly important skill in the real world. The grading process itself might thereby become a major teaching device rather than remain a source of anxious failure, indifference, or unrealistic pride.

A change process begun through several such intense experiences would have to be incorporated into the regular routine of school life if it were to produce lasting influence. For a time this would involve increased stress for all concerned as the new ways of relationship and new sharing of responsibility were explored. Such short-term dislocations could be justified, however, in terms of the long-range objectives of the undertaking; that is, the involvement of adolescents in responsibility for real decisions in the real world, their inclusion in planning the style and content of their own education, and their exposure, by adult example, to emotionally open and honest relationships with other people. Rather than any abdication of adult responsibility, what is contemplated here is an attempt by adults to demonstrate to adolescents the full meaning of the concept of responsible behavior. The Leader Lab experience suggests that when a faculty has available the necessary resources, and the time to work at developing these new relationships with one another and with the young people, a whole new dimension of education is opened for exploration.

REFERENCES

Friedenberg, E. Z. *Coming of age in America*. New York: Random House, 1965.
Schein, E. H., & Bennis, W. G. *Personal and organizational change through group methods*. New York: Wiley, 1965.

CHAPTER 13

Synanon: A Challenge to Middle-Class Views of Mental Health

John B. Enright

A cultivated man, wise to know and bold to perform, is the end to which nature works, and the education of the will is the flowering and result of all this geology and astronomy.—From the essay "Power" by Ralph Waldo Emerson.

A personal introduction seems necessary to place what I want to say in context. I have identified myself as a psychologist, either student or professional, for about twenty years, mostly in clinical research. Although I have done considerable practical and theoretical work communicating about psychology across class, ethnic, and language barriers, and thus have faced some of the problems of psychologists working in community mental-health programs, I am not presently involved directly in any such programs.

I have been a member of the Synanon Club of San Francisco for a year and a half as of fall 1967. This has been the most exciting personal adventure of my adult life, and perhaps some of this feeling will be communicated. I have learned a great deal that is "not dreamed of in our psychology," and I have begun to give what I did know from psychology deeper roots in my whole life instead of letting it exist in a semidetached, unassimilated way. I am intimately involved in the nonresident Synanon Club, and have held various offices in it.

Not surprisingly, this double identification has been occasionally confusing while writing this paper. I found myself saying *we* sometimes to mean "we psychologists" and other times to mean "we Synanists." The latter usage seemed to predominate; therefore, an unmodified *we* will refer to Synanon. Nothing I say should be construed as an official Synanon position; I speak strictly for myself, and indeed look forward to the necessity to defend in games[1] everything I say here.

I will attempt in this chapter to convey something of what the social movement called Synanon is like, why it is so difficult for professionals to grasp, and what its existence has to say about "community mental health." Some of these statements will sound harsh, and they are. I believe that mental-health professionals, even when well-meaning and competent by professional standards, have done great harm to many dope fiends.[2] By promising a cure they could not deliver, and by being so easily manipulated, professionals have at best prolonged and often increased the dope fiend's difficulties. If I can say something which will prevent these mistakes from being continued and extended to other community groups, I will consider this chapter a success. The body of this chapter was written in the fall of 1967. Factual or numerical statements refer to that time. There have been some developments and modifications of technique since then and some organizational changes, but nothing that requires extensive revision.

Synanon developed late in the 1950's out of the struggle of one man, Charles E. Dederich, to develop a way of life and a form of interaction with others that would enable him to stop drinking without spending all his energy in that one negative act. The early members who shared a hand-to-mouth existence with Dederich ("Chuck") were almost all long-time criminal dope fiends with big habits and long police records who had heard about Synanon in prison or on the street from others like them. Early in the 1960's Synanon began to receive national magazine publicity, and as a result, more middle-class addicts, some with college educations, began to appear at Synanon's door. Since then, there has been a steady broadening of membership in Synanon, and now a sizable minority of resident members have come in with a variety of difficulties in living other than addiction.

[1]The game, a form of small-group interaction developed in Synanon, will be described in detail in a later section.

[2]"Dope fiend" is the Synanon term for people who use dope and behave like fiends. Most of them outside of Synanon prefer to be called "drug addicts," as this sounds nicer, and hints that they have an illness for which they are not responsible.

Early in Synanon's development the club was supported almost entirely by small donations of money and goods and services from sympathetic and interested individuals in the community. Some of these people were interested in becoming more involved in sharing the wisdom and understanding of human behavior being developed by Synanon, and they were included sporadically and informally in Synanon activities. Finally in San Francisco in April 1966 their interest and involvement was formally recognized by the formation of the first of the Synanon "game clubs" in which nonresident members in large numbers could learn to play the Synanon game. Nonresidents are assumed to be functioning reasonably adequately in the community. They range from very marginally functioning individuals, for example, drunks and users of various "soft narcotics," to some highly successful in business or the professions. Individuals with histories of hard narcotic use are not permitted to join the nonresident club directly. As of fall 1967, the Synanon Club has about 1,000 resident members and 2,000 nonresidents, scattered among six major and several ancillary locations.

With its dynamic organization, 3,000 active members, and many more community friends and sympathizers, with its demonstrated competence in getting a number of dope fiends to stop shooting dope, and with a willingness to tackle any problem, Synanon would seem in a position to contribute a great deal to psychologists interested in community mental health. Already, its services have been used directly by some mental-health and corrections agencies, while others have modeled programs after it. However, throughout its history, Synanon has been an enigma and a headache to most behavioral scientists and professionals dealing with crime, delinquency, mental illness, welfare dependency, and other forms of misbehavior. Synanon has seemed unscientific and obscure, inadequately reporting its results. It has insulted well-meaning individuals in the professions, been considerably less than helpful to imitators, and seemed stiff-necked, suspicious, stubborn, and perverse. The mental-health professional will never understand Synanon so long as he tries to see it as simply an alternative approach to the common goal of mental health. There are significant differences between Synanon and the mental-health professions with respect to conceptions of the nature of the problem, the form of the solution, and the characteristic techniques employed.

Some of the crucial differences between Synanon and "mental-health" approaches can be summarized in a compact but complex phrase: Synanon does not *treat problems*, but rather *provides an opportunity for people*. This point is sometimes made almost over-dramatically in Synanon, when it is said that "Synanon cures dope addicts in one day; unfortunately it takes three years to eradicate thoroughly the cowardice, dishonesty, and ignorance that under-lay the dope habit." The problem as describable in the social setting in which it occurs disappears when it is placed in the Synanon situation. In its place appear in the individuals in question the fundamental human existential problems of responsibility, relatedness, courage, and meaningfulness. In Synanon's view, all of us are, to a rather serious extent, out of touch with ourselves and out of control of our own lives, lacking the courage, honesty, and awareness to live fully, responsibly, and effectively. Most of us, including those of us who are making out well by the world's standards, have nevertheless delegated vast areas of our human functioning to others—to specialists—and in turn become special-ists ourselves, developing narrower and narrower portions of our-selves more and more at the expense of the rest of our manhood and humanity. Economically, such specialization is very efficient; humanly, it is a destructive deadend. We have delegated our ag-gression to generals and prizefighters, our strength and competi-tiveness to athletes, our vivid sensuous experiences to the hippies, our sexuality to movie stars, and control of our own world to busi-nessmen and politicians. After such massive abdication of human responsibility for our own experiencing and functioning, it scarcely matters that some of us do not drink excessively or shoot dope.

Without these lost aspects of ourselves, we cannot become really solid, integrated people who can convert knowledge to wisdom and be fully honest with ourselves and others. We cannot take and hold firm moral positions and act as causal agents rather than as passive reactors in our worlds, living spontaneously and effectively with all our human equipment.

Thus Synanon is interested in people who are functioning in any way less than the fully human degree to which we are all capable. The particular form of irresponsibility or delinquency engaged in is not particularly important. It does not matter if we retreated into a dope haze, into an alcoholic fog, into a self-pitying depression, or into an intellectual vacuum. It does not matter if we acted out through stealing, income-tax evasion, impotence, or snobbery. Once a person is in the Synanon situation, the particular form of his previous misbehavior no longer matters. The *degree* of misbehavior does matter, and is recognized in the fact that some individuals are encouraged to become residents rather than nonresidents; but once in Synanon, there is little talk of the preexisting "symptom." Nor is there a "cure." The individual in Synanon engages in an increasingly exciting, involving, and fulfilling life. He gradually becomes an active agent in his own life, affecting other individuals and events to an increasing degree, at first in Synanon and later in the wider society. Whatever particular symptom he previously happened to exhibit as an alternative to leading this kind of life now becomes literally unthinkable. It is not that he "understands" why he did it or spends any great amount of energy in not doing it; simply as a byproduct of living an intensely human life, this symptom is sloughed off and disappears.

Synanon is not a treatment but an opportunity. If offers not a prescribed set of procedures resulting in predictable changes, but rather a structured situation within which the individual is permitted and encouraged to act in such a way as to recreate a more fully human life than the one he was leading before. This description follows from Synanon's historically respectable but currently unfashionable view that truth is to be created as much as discovered. The universe is not "out there" as a fully finished structure only waiting to be described by man, but rather is an unfinished, half-structured *opportunity* with which man must interact to create his own truth and reality. The personal and professional implications of this position are profound. Applied to a human life, this principle leads to the position that any individual, no matter how terrible his crimes or how miserable his current position, is not finished, determined, and fixed by his past. He can, if he wishes, at this moment begin in some small way to take charge of his life and to build a more satisfying one. It is not possible for the individual in Synanon to hide behind the pessimistic Freudian-scientific-deterministic view that "After all, it has all been decided since you were two years old, and little really can be done about it now." It is almost unbelievable and at times rather amusing how desperately people try to cling to some version of this view in order to avoid taking action in the present. It is perhaps most dramatic when the "hope-to-die-once-a-dope-fiend-always-a-dope-fiend" is faced with this position by individuals demonstrably similar to him, with equally "hopeless" pasts, but the same thing occurs to everyone in greater or lesser degree, as each of us is forced to struggle with the terrifying but liberating view that the past matters only in the way we use it in the present.

This philosophical principle also leads to some of the greatest difficulties that mental-health professionals have in understanding Synanon. If someone is providing a *treatment* for a *problem* he does undertake some responsibility for studying individuals for whom the treatment fails, or individuals with the problem who do not even undertake the treatment. Since Synanon offers an *opportunity*, it is not particularly interested in those individuals who elect not to avail themselves of it by not coming in the first place, or by dropping out ("splitting") after joining. It is totally uninterested in "background prognostic factors" as such. It does not select applicants or predict success in any objective, scientifically respectable way. After all, applicants select Synanon, and success is up to them. So treatment, in the sense of outcomes, cure rate, and so forth, cannot be evaluated. *There are no cures because there is no treatment.* Synanon is very interested in the new applicant's current attitude and willingness to work, which will be evaluated by a number of hard-nosed experts, whose "expertise" follows from their having been themselves in this desperate situation. But there is little or no selection in terms other than what the applicant himself brings. Synanon people describe the opportunity, make it a little difficult to achieve entry, and stand back.

The behavioral scientist is quite disturbed by this position, and says in effect, "But you aren't going about this right (that is, *our* way) so that we can evaluate you and compare you with all the other treatments for drug addiction." Synanon answers, "We aren't treating addicts. If you want to get to know what we *are* doing, come and see us and get acquainted as a human being. If not, go whine to each other in your journals, but don't waste our time." The "scientific" view that bad prognostic indicators really do operate, that individuals with these backgrounds *therefore* have less of a chance to change is a deeply rooted one in the professions, and is profoundly destructive. This view underlies the fact that most professional treatment of drug addiction fails. Professional and patient alike have a tacit understanding that the whole business is a farce since the patient is hopeless. With this assumption, it scarcely matters what is done. Many, probably a majority, of Synanon members have had one or more destructive contacts with this point of view, and it is this experience with professional-scientific pessimism that underlies some of Synanon's antiprofessional bias. Truth is created rather than discovered. Had Chuck Dederich and some of the early members of Synanon known that drug addiction was hopeless, or had there been a competent statistician around publishing his findings in the early days, Synanon would never have come into existence. By acting as if the task of getting dope fiends to stop shooting dope was possible in the face of all evidence to the contrary, the feat became possible. It is quite possible that some programs run by professionals to "cure drug addicts" will succeed. If so, in a quite fundamental way they will owe their success to the fact that Synanon broke the barrier of pessimism and hopelessness surrounding this social problem.

It is difficult to convey, particularly to professionals, what Synanon is all about, since it does not fit readily into easily available categories. Is it a social movement? Yes, but without a social goal that can be readily stereotyped. Is it a utopian movement? Yes, but it remains intimately entwined with the larger environment. Is it a therapy? Yes, but it denies categorically the value of illness concepts of misbehavior. Is it a form of recreation? Yes, indeed. It is an exciting and fulfilling way to spend time and may be the greatest entertainment bargain in present-day America. It is all of these, but not only these. I will try to convey very briefly something about Synanon by presenting it successively as a philosophy, a community, a technique, and as people.

THE SYNANON PHILOSOPHY

The first of Synanon's fundamental philosophical positions has already been implied in the above discussion. This is that it is possible to create a set of attitudes and feelings through action, rather than waiting for action to follow from feelings and attitudes. The most immature new dope fiend in Synanon knows at least intellectually some of the roles of an adult even if he has seldom put them into action. In Synanon he is expected to *act-as-if*—to act out some of these roles and to go through some of the motions he knows—no matter how strongly his feelings go against this kind of action. During the few hours a day that he is working in Synanon, he is expected to "shove his feelings in a corner" and do his job. Socializing with other people, he is expected to act-as-if he is a grown-up human being—again no matter how little he feels like it. As will be described later, there are places in the Synanon situation where he does not have to do this, but it is considered one of the most fundamental tools of growing up: to act grown-up, and let the attitudes and feelings follow from this. For the nonresident, acting-as-if might be used by a husband who has, say, been philandering before joining the club. He, too, will be expected to act-as-if he is a good husband, no matter how little he feels like it, and to deal in the game with the feelings he no longer acts out. It is not expected that acting-as-if on the basis of sheer will power can carry a person indefinitely, but he is expected to use it to the fullest extent possible as a tool, while new feelings and attitudes are developing underneath this action—feelings that later on he will be able to act on freely and spontaneously.

A second position, in almost paradoxical contrast to the above, is that any action a person takes, on whatever basis, is to be done as fully as possible with total commitment. Halfway measures, "good enough," "trying," are not acceptable. With each effort the individual runs into his inner reservations, which are reflected in behavior as holding back. He and others around him are alert to these reservations, to root them out and expose them and explore them. Some turn out to be invalid and are destroyed; some on examination seem to have validity. This information is fed back into action, and the individual changes the direction of his effort to fit with this new information, and again tries to act with total commitment on the new direction. The result of all this activity is that Synanon and its members often seem contradictory, to act by fits and starts, and to be quite inconsistent. This position is, however, quite consistent with what Ralph Waldo Emerson had to say in his essay on self-reliance: " ... speak what you think today in words as hard as cannon balls, and tomorrow speak what tomorrow thinks in hard words again, though it contradict everything you said today." Through this constant insistence on total commitment, the inner reservations and holdouts that most of us carry around for our entire lives are gradually exposed and used. Effectiveness of action increases, and by a series of successive approximations the individual gradually, if rather jerkily, moves into the course of life that is most truly consistent with his entire self.

A third fundamental principle of the Synanon philosophy is self-reliance. Part of the meaning of this term is that true "security," insofar as it is possible at all, can be found only within the self. To the extent that we lean on other people, money, status, title, or specialized knowledge, we are weak and at some level frightened. The other part of the meaning of this term is that such support really is available from within the individual, and that he only needs to learn to find and trust what is there. This part of the Synanon philosophy is based heavily on the writings of Emerson, and is perhaps best summarized in his essay on self-reliance:

He who knows that power is in the soul, that he is weak because he has looked for good out of him and elsewhere, and, so perceiving, throws himself unhesitatingly on his thought, instantly rights himself, stands in the erect position, commands his limbs, works miracles; just as a man who stands on his feet is stronger than a man who stands on his head.

Many of the "techniques" of Synanon that will be described later in this chapter can be understood as maneuvers to strip the individual of external support just as he is getting comfortable leaning on it and to force him to trust what comes from within, whether it seems sufficient at the moment or not. Thus, one of the characteristic features of the Synanon game is the convention that the individual is always totally alone in the game, with all friendships, titles, and status temporarily set aside and left at the door.

A fourth tenet that seems almost contradictory to the above is the almost Taoist notion of "letting it happen." The self which must be relied on is not only the narrow, conscious, planning ego, but the wider, more inclusive self; and although at times behavior can be driven by the conscious ego, at other times the individual or group must relax conscious control and trust what evolves naturally.

A fifth position in the Synanon philosophy is that there must somehow be room for all of a man somewhere. Our society has become seriously narrowed to verbal-rational activities and values. Room must be made for irrationality, for the comic, for aggression. There must be a place for deep communal feelings and for gossip, for guilt and for self-righteousness, for self-transcendence and for practical jokes—literally, for the sublime and for the ridiculous. Rational verbal activity must take its place as only one of many modes of human being.

From this position it follows that much that must be learned by human beings cannot be fully communicated in a rational-verbal way, and Synanon stresses the importance and centrality of *experiential learning*. Some knowledge is "in the gut" and cannot be communicated through words. Verbalizations about such knowledge are exactly that, and no more. Thus, many of the crucial events in Synanon are just that—events—and any attempts to communicate their impact verbally will be weak. The events can only be pointed at in context to be understood. Naturally, from this position it follows that much of what occurs in Synanon is manipulating people into positions where they will experience what they need to know in a preverbal way. Frequently, the individual subjected to this kind of positioning can later put into words what he has learned from it, but what he has learned could not have been successfully communicated to him through words before the experience. This takes place both inside and outside of the game. I will draw an example from a game. A woman gradually gave in to group pressure and finally admitted that she should take a certain step she had been rejecting for a long time. Instantly, the entire roomful of people reversed itself and pronounced her crazy to consider doing anything as silly as to take that step she had just agreed to. That phase of the game ended with the woman in tears of frustration, through which she learned beyond all telling how truly her choices in life were hers alone.

THE SYNANON COMMUNITY

For the resident it is an understatement to call Synanon a community. It is essentially another family. The resident failed in his first family to grow up in a way that permitted him to lead a good life. In Synanon he has the rare chance, a second family, to do it right. Synanon is quite clear in the extent to which the community becomes a family for the new member, and demonstrates this recognition by forbidding the new member to see his original family for several months. It might be more accurate to call Synanon an extended family or even a tribe, since there are many more people than in a normal family.

The community provides a network of relationships with people who are individuals to *react to* and *identify with*. A young man entering Synanon, for example, will find older people to respect, identify with, rebel against, and rage at; peers to love and compete with; and younger people whom he can haze and for whom he can become a guide and a teacher, solidifying what he learns and making it more real by giving it away to someone else. The tribe provides a wide variety of people to identify with and learn from. Some seem very close to him; some seem very far ahead. Throughout the whole chain or network of role models, however, he sees no totally unbridgeable gap. The professional-client gap, so difficult to cross, does not exist in Synanon. Since the tribe is a close, face-to-face community, living and working together, the models in the environment are available as *whole* people, not as fragmented, part-functioning people each of whom is seen in only a narrow, selected way. Rather, the people the individual selects as role models are visible to him in their entire range of functioning.

In such a community, with so many role models available and highly visible, it seems possible to form richer and more appropriate *identities*. The individual can pick and choose people who seem to fit with his developing potentials and take a little from each, putting together a more individualized and solid identity than is possible for most people in the wider culture. No longer does he have to tailor himself and his potentials drastically to fit the few models that are available to him. He can instead develop the parts of himself he does best and finds most valuable into a combination that is uniquely him. And since in the Synanon community, people are not defined only by their economic function, but rather by their whole humanity, there is simply more room for more different facets of people.

For the nonresident, the Synanon community is not as close or as intense as it is for the resident, but still for many it is the most involving community they have—a place to express themselves, to do and be things that are not possible elsewhere. In addition to the game, a nonresident will find available to him seminars, parties, fund-raising projects, work crews, conventions, staff and committee meetings, general sociability, speaking engagements, and a variety of interest and recreational groups. People who become closely involved usually bring in friends and acquaintances, and find themselves involved in Synanon with neighbors, co-workers, tradesmen, students, patients, teachers, and a variety of others with whom they also have contact in the wider environment. For some nonresidents, it is now possible to live directly in the Synanon situation as "resident nonresidents," renting apartments or homes from Synanon.

Another function of the community, one of central importance, seems especially alien and threatening to the pseudo-liberated middle-class American, with the exaggerated emphasis on privacy that we have developed. Most people do not seem able to *know clearly* and *live within* their own moral systems by themselves. Most of us engage in enough rationalized cheating—fudging income-tax returns, extending coffee breaks, trying a little marijuana, keeping a mistress, or outright stealing—that we are left with a chronic sense of unease, and are then vulnerable to moral pressure from others. The web of distortions necessary to conceal these derelictions interpersonally blocks intimacy and socially leaves us unable to act firmly, rightly, and righteously when necessary. Left to himself, a man too easily begins to lie to others and eventually to himself. Increasingly he says one thing while doing another, until he is out of touch with what is going on. He can know the full truth about himself and his actions only if he opens himself up to important people in his community, telling the truth to them and hearing it from them. In the Synanon game, the world's greatest experts on lying and rationalizing bring intense pressure on him simply to tell the truth in a situation in which the truth will have no secondary consequences.

Both the dope fiend and the respectable citizen only slowly and reluctantly give up their dirty little secrets. The rationalizer seems to feel that if he tells the truth, he will lose what little gratification he is getting. Instead, as he exposes his sources of discomfort or guilt, he can lay to rest finally those sources that are truly past and begin to take action on those still current. Some of the behavior he has been feeling guilty about he finds he can choose to give up. Some he finds he can modify, while some he can develop the courage to defend against the pressure of the group and thereafter continue without guilt. Thus he begins to define a moral posture that is truly his, open to view and convertible into behavior. Later he begins to reinforce this posture by exposing his story to others in the game, to encourage and support their efforts to do the same. Almost as a byproduct of this process the individual becomes more capable of easy and undefensive closeness with others. Intimacy, so elusive when sought directly (as in the currently fashionable encounter group), turns out to be a casual byproduct gotten, as it were, with the left hand while working directly toward the development of honesty and courage. This easy intimacy between people who share the game and the Synanon situation for a few years accounts in part for the pervasive sense of love and concern that is so immediately evident to the visitor to the Synanon community. In spite of the criticism, the bitter confrontations in games, the "squealing" on each other, the harsh treatment of the member who slips, and the merciless pressure toward the truth—or rather because of all these—a sense of caring for each other and the satisfaction of shared hard work are the dominant feelings among Synanon people.

The resident of Synanon submits himself more fully to the discipline of the group, surrendering his useless autonomy for a while, while he works toward an eventual more authentic autonomy. The nonresident retains direct control over his own life and puts himself to a lesser extent under the moral pressure of the group until that point when he begins to realize the liberating and growth-enhancing effect of telling the truth about himself and places himself more and more in the way of feedback from those around him. Those of us who have become deeply involved as nonresidents almost always make sure that we bring friends, co-workers, and others in our life circle into the club with us, to make ourselves open to feedback and exposure. In this frame of reference, it is almost obligatory for an individual who knows something potentially important about another member to pass this on, so that the individual can be confronted with it. Plain, simple gossip becomes a valuable tool in the Synanon situation. The individual who does something dishonest harms himself; the individual who knows this and does not confront the other person with it harms himself, the other person, and to some extent the whole group. The story of "cop-out night," when the Synanon members who had been cheating and using a little of various chemicals on the side finally brought their own and their friends' dishonesty out in the open, and stopped it, epitomizes this attitude.

THE SYNANON TECHNIQUE

The most basic, powerful, and novel technique developed in Synanon is the *game*. Without the game the Synanon situation would probably cease to exist within a couple of months. However, it is important to point out that without the rest of the environment to provide structure and context, the game could not be played as it is. Professionals looking at the Synanon situation often notice the game first as being the most salient feature, forming a "figure" against the background of the rest of the situation. It is only when seen out of context this way that the game bears even a superficial relationship to group therapy.

In the game, from 10 to 15 Synanon members meet, usually on Synanon property. At least a few are fairly experienced in playing the game. There are two rules: (1) no violence or threats of violence and (2) no consciousness-distorting chemicals. Games may last anywhere from one to twenty-four hours. The most common length is 2½ to 3½ hours. Rarely, if ever, will exactly the same people meet in a game. Typically, an individual will be playing a game with a few people who were in a previous game with him, a sprinkling of totally new people, and some he remembers from previous games but not in the recent past. Within these broad limits, almost anything can and does happen. The whole range of human experience is possible. Players try, among other things, to tell the truth about themselves and others as best they can. Attack and defense, dominance struggles, catharsis, ridicule, sympathy, projection, identification, confrontation are all part of the game. An attempt is made to create crises and emergencies, to drive people to the end of what they know and hopefully past that point, to force action where no action seems possible. An attempt is made to strip away every mask that is put on, knock off every hat that is donned, and drive a person out of every position he takes. A man is basically always alone in a game; all friendships are left at the door, as well as all status and titles. Alliances are fleeting and ad hoc, and when the purpose of one alliance is finished, the most likely subject next raised in the game will be that very alliance. In a good game there is an abundance of comedy. "The epic is reduced to a gag, and the momentary lapse of awareness is magnified to a crime against humanity." In the game, people work through their disagreements, express their negative affects, carry out their quarrels and dominance struggles, let off steam, make the first tentative exploration of new parts of themselves, and express feelings that are unfamiliar.

The most important function of the game is to permit all the above to happen *there,* so that it does not happen elsewhere. In the rest of the Synanon environment, the Synanon member is always cooperative, does his job no matter how he feels, is civil at all times, responsible, constructive, positive, and controlled—acting-as-if he is a mature human being whether he feels like it or not. The tensions engendered in a dope fiend who does that for more than a few hours can then be discharged in a game. Thus the relationship between the game and the environment is in part one of *polarization*. Between the two, all sides of life can be fully expressed. The necessary business of running the Synanon Corporation and carrying out the business of life can be done smoothly, uncontaminated by petty rivalries and dominance struggles that are part of human living. In the resident situation, if a man whose job is to scrub toilets gets angry at his boss because he feels he is being overworked, he nonetheless behaves himself on the job. He then may "call a game" on his boss in which the boss has to leave all status advantages behind and face him man-to-man. If by any chance the boss should try to carry his anger outside the game and get revenge on the job, this would immediately be a subject for another game. A husband and wife in the nonresident situation who have been quarreling seriously can use the situation in the same way: "acting-as-if," behaving themselves, and being courteous at home, and using the game—and extra games if need be— to "dump their garbage" and to make their complaints. For individuals, resident or nonresident, who have rather undifferentiated affective lives, often not knowing exactly how they feel and acting rather impulsively, this polarization between game and environment is a priceless opportunity to begin learning differentiation, to learn what kinds of feelings to hold back and what kinds to express. As indicated, there is room for all of life in the whole situation, but there is an insistence on appropriateness, on saving some feelings for some places and others for others. The long-range goal of this approach is to produce people who can express any feeling at any time; but on the way to this final integration, differentiation and separation are crucial.

To maintain the polarity of game and environment, two additional boundary rules are necessary about the relationship of these two elements. One is "When it's over, it's over." The game has its own reality; nothing is to be carried out literally and used. A friend or wife or co-worker is obligated to attack as vigorously as possible in the game, and the subject of this attack understands that, although very real at the moment, this does not apply to all of life, and a friendly relationship can and should be resumed on the way out the door. Incidentally, part of the environmental context of the game for nonresidents is a social hour after games to allow for "picking up," socialization, and reestablishing possibly ruptured ties. The existence of this "pick-up" allows the game to have more impact. A person can be left in a rather shaken state in a game—a state that is sometimes necessary for learning—with a recognition that an experienced game player will make sure that after the game normal relations are reestablished and the person left with the awareness that what was attacked was his behavior and not himself.

The other boundary rule between game and environment is "Don't play the game outside the game." As much as possible, unless there is some immediate need for a "pull-up" in the environment, any kind of criticism or negative affect should be saved for a game and the confrontation made there instead of in the environment.

The game and the environment meet in two ways: through the *indictment* and the *motion.* In the indictment, some piece of behavior or action on the part of an individual, usually from the environment, is brought into the game. The individual is confronted with some real behavior; perhaps he was ten minutes late to an appointment, perhaps he left a dirty coffee cup in a previous game, or perhaps he behaved unpleasantly at work or at a Synanon party. The behavior can be large or small, of obvious importance or apparent triviality. Nonetheless, this is the typical starting point of the game. The indictment is presented usually in mordant and righteous tones, and often in outrageously exaggerated form. Immediately, others in the game join in with similar incidents or confirmations of the indictment and begin to weave a pattern around the indicted individual. He may attempt immediately to justify or defend, and in this defense he may reveal the seeds of a new indictment. This will be picked up and developed, and the game is thoroughly under way.

Frequently, when an individual has been the subject of attention in a game for some time and the others are in some sense finished with him, he will be left with a "motion." The motion is a prescribed activity which can be extremely simple, like dressing in a certain manner, or more extensive. Fundamentally, it is a set of activities that the individual is supposed to engage in, not necessarily understanding why nor expecting any particular result, with the expectation that by engaging in this activity he will position himself to perceive his world differently and elicit different responses from it. A motion is not advice in the usual sense, but rather an experiment the individual is encouraged to perform, acting some behavior "as if" in order to open the way for changes in attitude or feeling.

The game has been described in quite general terms so far. It is important to emphasize that it takes a wide variety of different specific forms depending upon the particular purpose of the game and the level of experience of the people playing it. Some games have a serious, "heavy" tone; some, particularly when played by newcomers, are noisy and angry. Many times the game will seem like an absurd and hilarious spoof. The game is not particularly designed to *solve* problems, but rather to *demolish* them—to shatter all the perceived elements of a problem and reassemble them into a new form. Usually, once a problem has been clearly stated, either it can be solved almost immediately or it turns out to be insoluble; rather than reworking some tired old formulation of a problem, the game will try to position the person differently in his life so that the problem changes form and becomes perhaps a new problem, perhaps an opportunity, perhaps no problem at all. Whenever Synanon is in a state of crisis, the first response usually is to turn inward and play the game—not as a problem-solving procedure or as a "brainstorming" session, but rather as an opportunity for the people involved to discover where they truly are emotionally, and to begin working from that point. The game has changed in many ways since the early days of Synanon, and often seems different in different installations, depending on the dominant people in the installation. There is a different quality to the game as played by nonresidents compared with residents. However, despite all the surface differences, the game remains the game, and remains Synanon's most important technique.

Synanon has many other environment-structuring and behavior-modifying techniques, much too numerous to go into detail about here. A few of these are the morning meeting, the noon seminar, the cerebration, the probe, the haircut, the dissipation, the trip, and the stew. Some of these have been described in Yablonsky (1965); others have been formulated since the publication of that book. In terms of detailed techniques, Synanon is in a constant state of flux, with new procedures constantly being created, modified, and destroyed in favor of other methods. What is most important about Synanon is not specific techniques but its openness to the whole range of human wisdom about change in human behavior. Dynamic psychiatry has taken a few tools of change (for example, insight, acceptance, and rational analysis) and honed and developed these to maximum efficiency. However, at the same time, it has left many other tools to rust, unused. The tools that have been developed in dynamic psychiatry are efficient only within certain contexts with certain kinds of people. For most people, extensive change cannot be achieved without all of the methods that can possibly be brought to bear. Synanon recognizes the value of rationality, analysis, insight, and acceptance, but only as parts of a much more extensive pattern. Synanon is somehow able to make use of human motives and behaviors that are almost totally omitted from the repertoire of dynamic psychiatry.

This is perhaps most obvious in Synanon's ability to deal with, and turn to good account, human aggression and hatred. These are accepted as inevitable parts of human nature, and a place is provided—primarily, but not only, in the game—for their expression and harnessing. A good Synanist is highly skillful at mobilizing and directing aggression and putting it to work. I have seen a skilled Synanist in a matter of two or three minutes criticize a newcomer viciously for a job poorly done, thus transmuting the newcomer's vague guilt into intense anger focused on the Synanist. The anger was then turned back onto the newcomer and focused particularly on his poor behavior. The Synanist then praised him for something else, and left him steamed up, mad at his own ineptness, and determined to correct it. Most of us in the mental-health professions would be incapable of taking the necessary step of developing anger and risking that it be focused on ourselves. Certainly in my own practice before joining Synanon, I found it impossible to accept and use strong anger, but had to turn it aside or "analyze" it, taking myself as a human being out of the relationship. The tolerance, or rather enthusiastic acceptance, of aggression as a part of human life enters into many of the techniques Synanon has developed that are almost inaccessible to mental-health disciplines.

Although it has already been touched upon, the use of role modeling deserves additional mention here as one of Synanon's most powerful techniques. A Synanon motto is: "You can only teach what you are," and this is deliberately and consciously used to the hilt in Synanon, where people are actively urged to seek and define role models. Powerful use is also made of the fact that *being* a role model is a most effective way to bind a person to a course of behavior that is best for him. When he begins to feel a little shaky and not sure that it is worth it, a look around at people who are looking up to him is sometimes the best way to keep himself on the track over a difficult period. I emphasize this technique of Synanon because it is the one most lacking in the professional-client relationship. Quite often, a mental-health professional does not let himself appear as a full human being to the client, but rather hides behind technique and the safety of his professional role. Even those exceptions who can permit themselves to be open can have less than optimal effect since the client sees them as being in unattainable positions. In the mental-health professions, we create and maintain a massive barrier against our being effective, and our hardest efforts at best only neutralize rather than overcome this barrier.

THE SYNANON PEOPLE

Synanon's product is people "with their heads screwed on straight," and the final test of its efficacy lies in the quality of these people. People who have been around Synanon long enough to be thoroughly affected by its dynamic are, just as people, rather exceptional. Considering the typical Synanon member's background of crime, narcotics, and/or prostitution, his current effectiveness is remarkable. Not always particularly "well-adjusted," and often quite prickly, they are people who know what they want and are actively getting it, but at the same time leading lives that are morally sound and showing consideration for others important to them. They are living evidence of the effectiveness of Synanon and powerful arguments against the plaint of problem-ridden people who want to give up "because I had such a bad childhood."

Most of the inner-core group of Synanon, people who have been around for a long time and are deeply involved, are people who had in the past led lives of violence—violence that is now controlled and transmuted into a vigorous directness that is exciting and challenging. This fact about Synanon may be what is responsible for the qualitative difference between the Synanon ideal and the middle-class view of mental health. I think Emerson had the "mentally healthy" middle-class individual in mind when he wrote, "We are parlor soldiers; the rugged battle of fate where strength is born we shun." It is ironic that the nineteenth-century's middle-class ideals, as formulated by Emerson, are finally being implemented by this century's lower class. It is small wonder that this century's middle class has a little difficulty understanding the phenomenon!

SYNANON AND COMMUNITY MENTAL HEALTH

The description of Synanon in this chapter has been brief and sketchy. More information is available in published form (see the References at the end of this chapter), and more is forthcoming. As has already been suggested, there is a limit to what can be communicated about Synanon verbally, and it is strongly recommended that anyone interested come down in person and get acquainted. There is no chance at all of grasping what Synanon is about, without meeting some Synanon people and experiencing the atmosphere first-hand.

Synanon has something to offer community mental health both practically and theoretically. Practically, Synanon as it exists today is prepared to accept people from all parts of the community, with almost any "community mental-health problem." As indicated, little attention will be paid to the problem as such, but the *people* are welcome. A certain amount of motivation—often in the form of desperation—is necessary to get people over the threshold. Once in the Synanon setting, where their social problem is transmuted to an existential one, people who previously seemed almost hopelessly mired down can develop surprising strength and motivation and make use of the Synanon setting.

A second immediately available practical use of Synanon is through its people. Many community mental-health programs might find considerable use for a few tough, wise, and self-reliant people, well-equipped to deal with hostility and aggression, and frequently from similar backgrounds to those of the "clients" involved, to act as role models and change agents. Attempts to do this in the past have sometimes run into bureaucratic difficulties over associating with ex-addicts or paying Synanon for its people. Additionally, at times Synanon has felt it necessary to withdraw from some programs for the sake of its own or its people's development. The possibility exists, however.

A third use of Synanon is the one I personally am making. Mental-health professionals ("shrinks") have, among Synanon members, a reputation for being passive, evasive, afraid of anger, and certainly the most easily conned of all professionals. (I have heard oldtime members, far enough from the street to be permitted such reminiscences, chuckle about dragging out a withdrawal for a month, while getting high-quality drugs for it from a sympathetic psychiatrist.) Most of this stereotype fits me only too well. I have, in the Synanon situation, become far more able to act, to say what I mean to anyone about anything without becoming evasive or compromising. I am learning to get out from behind the shield of my professional role and to face people from all walks of life man-to-man. For the mental-health professional about to embark on a community mental-health program with people quite different from himself, I can imagine no better training ground in toughness and flexibility than the Synanon situation.

Synanon "techniques" resist transplanting quite stubbornly, and attempts to copy Synanon in any mechanical way usually fail. However, I have found it possible, having absorbed the Synanon philosophy, to apply *it* to a different situation, letting new forms develop that are fitting to the new situation, yet faithful to Synanon's philosophical tenets. I have done things in a mental-hospital setting and in private practice that I consider to be direct applications of Synanon, though they do not resemble any Synanon "technique" directly. This is yet another way in which the interested professional can make good use of Synanon.

At present, however, Synanon can be of only small-scale practical help with existing problems. Far more important are the questions it raises and the answers it implies about the middle-class professional member of the Establishment who attempts to achieve some results with a group of people from a different background who are exemplars of some social problem. What can we learn from the fact that professional efforts to "work with" drug addicts have been a large-scale failure, while Synanon has had a small but solid success? I would like to look briefly at this contrasting success and failure with the hope of discovering some general points that would help a professional contemplating a community mental-health program.

Briefly and bluntly, we professionals have failed with drug addicts because we do not know enough, are not men enough, do not care enough, and are not hopeful enough. The body of psychological assumptions, theories, and techniques commonly available to the average practitioner is simply not adequate to deal with the average dope fiend. The skill and knowledge of the mental-health professional are tied to certain conditions, and are applicable primarily to people like him, with similar middle-class problems and limitations. We professionals do not seem capable of broadening and extending our knowledge outside of these limits. The knowledge we need is not technical but human; we do not need more facts, but to *be* wise, tough, and honest. Most mental-health professionals are pathetic putty in the hands of a street-wise dope fiend. Quite simply, professionals are not men enough to do the job. Professionals do not understand or empathize with dope fiends, and the dope fiends in turn are quite uninterested in identifying with or learning from the professional. He has his own hangups and problems that quite often are not similar to those that trouble the dope fiend, and he really does not seem to care about his "client." His own natural concerns—of his job, his living, his publications, and his status among his peers—often seem to conflict directly with those of the dope fiend. The dope fiend, having been shucked by experts, knows a hustle when he sees one, and senses at some level that he is an object to the professional, and a hopeless object at that. The professional "knows" that dope fiends are an intractable and incurable lot. He may occasionally be deluded into thinking he has a curable one on his hands, but his underlying expectation is one of failure—an expectation generally shared by the dope fiend. The dope fiend, therefore, exploits the professional for drugs, privileges, and for his own amusement, while the professional exploits the dope fiend as a job, as a topic for a publication, and as an object of pity and contempt.

These are harsh words, but they must be heard if we professionals are to profit from our serious mistakes and not perpetuate them with other problem groups. I would like to end by formulating a series of questions to be asked of each community mental-health professional as he comtemplates or engages in any kind of community mental-health program on any target population. The questions are the ones posed to me by Synanon's successful existence; they are provocative and challenging—perhaps even unpleasant —but they must be heard and should be answered.

1. Whose ends are you serving in this program? Yours? Society's?

Those of science? The client's? Naturally, goals will be mixed and complex, and some will be "selfish," but it is extremely important to be clear with yourself and others. If part of the purpose of the program is to pacify and placate a population so that the middle class can sleep better, *say so.* If part of the purpose is to generate a publication or get a grant, *say so.* If part of the purpose is to create in yourself a glow of helpfulness, *say so.* If your program includes some mental-health goal for the target population, does it fit? Does it really make sense to and for these people, or does it merely make you more comfortable? Do you genuinely think the program will succeed?

2. Do you know, respect, and care for some members of your population *as people?* Can you set aside your professional props and get down ("relate") with them, touching their common humanity with yours? Can you share some interests and activities, maintaining your standards without offending theirs? Are you reasonably acceptable to them? Is there any quality important to people in your population that you are seriously lacking in, so that they would have a difficult time respecting you? How would you be as a role model for a client in your population? Would he be on the right track if he behaved as you do, or would this lead to more difficulties for him in his environment? If you would be acceptable as a role model, are you sufficiently available to him as a whole person so that he *could* model himself effectively after you? "You can only teach what you are." Are you satisfied with the lesson your life will teach?

To answer these questions is not easy, and is not a purely cognitive task. I am convinced, however, that success in a community mental-health program is crucially dependent on the answers to these questions.

This chapter has described Synanon, a nonprofessional organization in which people with severe character disorders have been able to make extensive changes in their conduct. Its philosophy, community, technique, and people have been described, as well as some of the difficulties that professionals have in understanding and accepting Synanon. The implications its success has for the middle-class professional conducting a community mental-health program are discussed, and from this a series of questions has been posed for the community mental-health professional.

REFERENCES

Casriel, D. *So fair a house.* Englewood Cliffs, N.J.: Prentice-Hall, 1963.

Endore, G. *Synanon.* New York: Doubleday, 1968.

Pamphlets published by Synanon: #1 *The human sport* by G. Endore; #2 *Outrageous impudence* by G. Endore; #3 *The perpetual stew* by G. Endore; #4 *The trip* by B. Harrison.

Yablonsky, L. *The tunnel back: Synanon.* New York: Macmillan, 1965.

CHAPTER 14

Client Participation
and Community Change

Joan Grant and J. Douglas Grant

1. Sentenced to prison for first-degree robbery at 23 following a series of supermarket holdups. Arrest record began at 13 on charges of petty theft and being a runaway. Subsequent arrests for burglary, drunkenness, and battery. Served one jail term. Raised in rural areas; family were agricultural workers. Quit school after the tenth grade. Work record as laborer was good but unstable. Gambling and frequent, excessive drinking have been problems.

2. Sentenced to prison for first-degree robbery at 22; paroled three years later. Sentenced to prison at 25 for attempted robbery of jewelry store during which was shot and nearly killed. Known delinquency since 14 when sent to reformatory for robbery. At 16 served term in state juvenile institution, also for robbery; at 21 spent five months in jail for assault. Raised in black ghetto communities. Completed high school at 18 while confined. No steady work since 20. Prior to last confinement was making a living by systematic robbery.

3. Sentenced to prison for first-degree robbery at 25; paroled three years later. Returned to prison within a year as parole violator for possession of heroin; reparoled three years later. Sentenced to prison six months later for possession of firearms by an ex-felon. Known delinquency since 13 when charged with burglary and malicious mischief. Has served jail terms for car theft and for possession of narcotics; frequent arrests for traffic violations, drunk driving, suspected burglary, and narcotics possession. Described by institution staff as a manipulator, incurably delinquent, and sure to be back in prison within two months. Raised in rural and then urban Mexican-American communities. Left ninth grade at 16, but continued schooling while confined. When not confined, has worked sporadically at unskilled jobs.

These men have been persistent problems to the community since an early age, and the community has responded by expelling them each time their behavior became too blatantly troublesome or deviant. They have spent significant portions of their youth in confinement, and a good part of both their formal and informal education has taken place in correctional institutions.

As this is written, these men have been out of prison, out of trouble, and working steadily for periods of from 2½ to 3 years. Their annual salaries range between $12,000 and $15,000. One is employed by a state antipoverty agency, where he works as a program developer for manpower-training programs; he is enrolled part-time in a community college. Another is employed by a private hospital as coordinator of a community mental-health program in which patients are developed as active participants in their own rehabilitation. The third is working as an evaluator of education programs for a federal agency and is employed part-time on the faculty of a state university where he serves as a resource person in the training of graduate students in criminology.

These men are part of a group of eighteen who participated in a demonstration project in 1965-1966. Twelve of the eighteen are working successfully in what can broadly be called program development. Their histories and work experiences are similar to those described above. Of the six not now working in this field, only one is confined.

This small-scale project raises some issues and suggests some ways in which community problems and problem people can be approached. The project is described briefly below. We will then consider its implications for what is called here community psychology.

THE NEW CAREERS DEVELOPMENT PROJECT [1]

To begin with, the project was not an experiment in individual rehabilitation. Our interest was in careers, not persons. We were concerned with the development of new sources of manpower in the human-service fields and with the processes necessary to bring about change in institutions to accommodate this new source. At that time, we were working in the crime and delinquency field,

[1] The project was sponsored by the Institute for the Study of Crime and Delinquency under a research grant (OM-01616) from the National Institute of Mental Health and was carried out with the cooperation of the California Department of Corrections. The opinions expressed here do not necessarily reflect those of any of these three organizations.

and we saw offenders and ex-offenders as a significant source of new manpower there, but the assumptions that underlay the project have much broader relevance. Briefly, this was the argument.

1. There are currently severe shortages of workers in the professional service fields, especially those of education, health, welfare, and corrections. Predicted estimates of future manpower needs in these fields (based upon both expected population increase and increased demands for service) indicate that these shortages will soon be critical.

2. Services as presently delivered are inadequate to meet the needs. Aside from the fact that there is not enough health, education, and welfare to go around and that what there is, is unequally distributed, services as they exist today are considered too costly and too ineffective. Complaints come from both the taxpaying public and the client recipients of service. The public complains that costs for services and in some cases clients themselves have gotten out of hand. Young people are neither educated nor quiet, delinquent and criminal acts are not adequately controlled, welfare and health cost too much and their use is being abused. On the other side, clients are becoming more vocal about the failure of public helping agencies to serve them and in some areas— notably education—the clients are organizing to take over part of the service functions themselves.

3. There is obvious need for change. Some federal money is available for research and demonstration in ways of improving service delivery, but much of this activity takes place peripherally to the everyday operation of service agencies. Within agencies the need for change is often recognized, but the development of new programs is generally left to staff who are occupied with the operation of existing programs and have neither the time nor the inclination for the task. A growing number of agencies have established special program-development or planning staffs whose sole function is the creation and implementation of new program ideas. This planning and development function should be much expanded, however, and should include the recipients of service in the planning function.

4. Even granted adequate funds and willingness to try new approaches, there is concern about the failure of professional workers to work effectively with, or even to reach, a significant

proportion of the client population. There are a number of examples (Alcoholics Anonymous and Synanon are two obvious ones) of programs in which nonprofessionals have been more effective in reaching problem people than have professionally trained staff. If this is true for a helping role, why not for program development? Might nonprofessionals not only fill a needed role for the helping professions, but also contribute something unique through their accessibility to client groups.

The New Careers Project was intended to test whether or not nonprofessionals (offenders) could be trained to fill program-development roles. When the study was conceived, these were seen as roles specifically in the crime and delinquency field. As the project and job opportunities developed, these were broadened to include program development in other areas of human service.

The Trainees

In the selection of participants for the project, no attempt was made to choose men who were representative of the prison population as a whole, since the aim was to demonstrate only that there is an untapped potential within the offender group. Selection was limited mainly by the requirements of the Department of Corrections. The department's concern about possible notoriety and embarrassment if a trainee should get into trouble led to the elimination of men whose commitment offenses were rape, child molesting, heroin use, or assault, and men with histories of severe mental illness or chronic alcoholism. Men had to volunteer for the program and, most importantly, had to be eligible for parole by the end of the training period, a condition that ruled out most applicants. Project interests led to choosing men only from the department's living-group (therapeutic-community) programs, on the grounds that experience in group living and group interaction would facilitate adaptation to the group-oriented training program. It was further required that the men read at least at the eighth-grade level, since the length of the program precluded any extensive remedial work. Men who met all these conditions were further screened for suitability through interviews by project staff and through ratings by other inmates in their living units.

The trainees were currently in prison on charges of robbery, burglary, forgery, and theft. Nearly half had been previously confined in juvenile or adult institutions. Their ages ranged from 22 to 35; their formal education, from ninth grade to a few months of college; and their IQ's on the Army General Classification Test from 98 to 123. According to the department's statistical prediction measure of parole behavior, 58 per cent were expected to be successful over a two-year period.

The project included a control group of nine men, selection conditions not permitting a larger number. Compared with the project participants, these men were slightly older, had more prior confinements but fewer aggressive offenses, and had a slightly lower predicted chance for success on parole. They were about the same as the experimental group in intelligence and reasonably similar in educational and occupational background. The two groups are compared in Table 1.

TABLE 1. CHARACTERISTICS OF EXPERIMENTAL AND CONTROL GROUPS

Characteristic	Experimental	Control
Number in group	18	9
Average age	26	31
Served prior prison term	2	5
Served prior juvenile term	7	5
Admission offense:		
First-degree robbery	5	3
Second-degree robbery	3	
Possession of firearms	1	
Grand theft	6	
Second-degree burglary	1	1
Forgery	2	3
Statutory rape		1
Marijuana sales		1
Average IQ (A.G.C.T.)	110	111
Completed high school	11	5
Past occupation:		
Sales, business	4	
Skilled labor		3
Semiskilled and unskilled labor	14	6
Member of minority group	8	3
Prediction of parole success	58%	52%

The Training Program

There were three groups of trainees, with some overlap among the groups as indicated below. Training was done at a state prison and lasted four months. The training program was built around a set of learning principles which can be summarized as a set of beliefs: that there should be freedom for different approaches to learning, that learning should be meaningful to the trainee, and that the trainee should be an active participant in it, that a study of oneself is important but should take place in the context of a task rather than a therapeutic orientation, and that involvement with, and commitments made to, one's peers may be more helpful in learning than is involvement in an authority-learner relationship.

To this end, we wanted maximum participation of the trainees both in planning and in carrying out the training curriculum; content centered around specific tasks or projects initiated by the trainees; self-study focused on the trainee's achievement of tasks; and maximum involvement of peers in providing feedback, counsel, and structure, as well as in the training process itself.

The training program was built around team activity, a team consisting of two trainees and a staff consultant. During the first training phase, a social-science graduate student worked with the team two days a week. Students were not available for Phases 2 and 3. During these phases each team was assigned an "older," a trainee graduate of Phase 1 who had not yet been paroled.

The scheduled training time occupied 57 hours a week, but the trainees worked far in excess of this. About half of their time was taken up with team projects. These were planned and carried out by the trainees themselves, with staff help given as it was requested. The projects in Phase 1 consisted of attitude surveys, using prison inmates and staff as subjects (for example, a survey to determine reasons for dropouts from the prison education program). These projects gave the trainees practice in preparing interview schedules, interviewing, conducting study groups, and coding data, as well as in writing proposals and reports. They were not, however, very closely related to the actual work that program-development assistants, as the trainees were called, were doing on the outside.

Using the experiences of the Phase 1 trainees working in the field, and consulting with state-agency staff, the Phase 2 and 3 trainees used inmate interviews and study groups to develop job descriptions and career ladders for nonprofessionals in the fields of criminal rehabilitation, alcoholism, medicine, and mental retardation. These projects were a substantial improvement over the attitude surveys of Phase 1. They were more specifically related to the concerns of the project, and they required the trainees to develop skills they were more likely to use later on. The team would begin by defining the unmet needs of the clients of the agency in question. They described functions that nonprofessionals might perform, and they assessed the problems of incorporating nonprofessional staff into the agency's existing structure. They gave some attention to training programs and career ladders that the agency might adopt.

Besides team projects, there were a number of total-group activities: study groups in research methods, in interviewing techniques, in group dynamics, and in organization change; seminars on writing and on current social trends and issues; self-study sessions concerned with the trainee's progress toward his avowed goals; planning and evaluation sessions concerning the project itself; and living-learning groups which dealt with problems of living and working together, of learning, and of concerns about the future. Aside from the living-learning groups, which met nightly, each activity occupied a two-hour weekly period and was planned and led by the trainees.

The Field Experience

When the New Careers Project was first conceived, we thought of the trainee as a kind of "linker," expediter, and communicator between client groups and program administrators. We saw his role as collecting data—ideas, feelings, behavior—about programs, especially from program participants, feeding these data back to program planners, and establishing some link between the two. This notion had been discussed with a number of persons in correctional agencies throughout the state, and we anticipated placements in this field for all the trainees. Intensive training was to continue following parole for at least four months, with reliance on the shared experience of the peer group, several of whom were expected to work in each of two or three geographic areas.

We were naive in this expectation, and we were in error. There is a gulf between the recognition by a staff member that his agency ought to change and his ability or even interest in bringing about the necessary changes in his organization. Anticipated jobs did not materialize, and the project faced a series of crises as each group of trainees was graduated and each temporary job was terminated.

The project director moved into a full-time job-development role. Using project funds directly to pay the trainees, developing contracts with other agencies for trainee services, using personal contacts across the country to develop jobs, and backing up these activities with an out-of-pocket loan fund, the men were maintained in reasonably steady employment. The jobs were short-term. Most of the outside funding came directly or indirectly from Office of Economic Opportunity programs. These programs often had uncertain funding, and payrolls were not always met on time. There was general uncertainty about how long programs would last. Money was a critical issue for both the project and the trainees throughout the first year of field experience.

The initial jobs fell roughly into two categories, training and program development. In the former, the project trainees served as trainers of the unemployed or economically marginal groups in programs designed to develop community organizers and parole aides. In the latter, the trainees conducted surveys of new career possibilities for the poor within public-service agencies and worked with staff of these agencies to help them define new entry-level jobs and to build appropriate career sequences from these.

Since the early months of training, both the trainees and the world outside have moved, and it is impossible to say what precise mixture of the two is responsible for their present success. Over this time period (29 to 44 months), the trainees have been employed in private social agencies, in nonprofit and in profit-making research and development organizations, in city, state, and federal government agencies, in county and state Offices of Economic Opportunity and community-action agencies, and in universities. Their salaries have risen from a starting point of $6,000 up to $15,000. They have worked in Washington, D.C., Alaska, California, Illinois, Nevada, New Jersey, New York, Oregon, and Washington. One group of trainees now constitutes the entire senior staff of a $1.5-million manpower program funded by the Department of Labor. While the informal contacts and the job-development work of the project director led to many of the placements, the trainees have gradually taken over the job-development role, both for themselves and for others, and are now in a position to hire the project director as an occasional consultant. While the jobs are still funded largely by "soft money," they are longer-term. Trainees now change jobs to improve their position, not because they have to. They are beginning to bring about change in the institutions with which they work. One group, for example, has worked out some new accreditation procedures with a community college for the work they themselves are doing as well as for the men they are training. Several are involved in developing organizations of nonprofessional workers in the human-service fields.

Of the six trainees not now working in the field, one was returned to prison and another walked off the job shortly after release on parole. The other four stayed with program-development work for a year and a half or more, when it became clear to them and sometimes to others that it was too much for them. One of the four is in college and the other three, as far as is known, are working at semiskilled laboring jobs.[2]

IMPLICATIONS OF THE NEW CAREERS PROJECT

We are living in a time in which increasing numbers of persons are becoming "outs," people for whom our culture has little or no use. These include most importantly the ghetto and rural poor, but they also include young people generally, the aged, and those stigmatized by mental or physical illness or by incarceration. They will probably soon also include the technologically dispossessed of the lower-middle class whose growing frustrations are beginning to be expressed politically.

We see these diverse groups linked by the needs for meaning, for belonging, and for participation. It is obvious that increased welfare payments, however needed and however distributed, are not going to touch the feelings of alienation and powerlessness that underlie much urban unrest and personal misery. Psycholo-

---

[2]Three of the trainees are failures in terms of the parole prediction measure, though one of these we now count a success. Four months after his parole he was returned to prison as a technical parole violator for becoming involved in a fight; he served seven months, then returned to program-development work. Of the other two, one was returned to prison on a new robbery conviction. The other disappeared shortly after his parole, but was later reinstated. He had not been involved in any delinquent activity but has not been in contact with the project since that time. This record (17 per cent failure) is considerably better than was expected. In contrast, the failure rate for the nine controls (three have been returned to prison and one has disappeared) is about what was predicted.

gists as well as others who try to move into the arena of community change must at some point—and preferably very soon—consider ways of giving a meaningful participant role to the targets of change.

The New Careers Project was a limited and crude attempt to utilize a participant approach in developing people to bring about change within social agencies. It is offered here neither as a model nor as a prescription. The experiences growing out of the project may be of some use to persons concerned with bringing about change in institutions and in the community.

The Professional's Role

We did not approach this project as psychologists. Most of our specific skills as psychologists were irrelevant. What we had to offer was a point of view, a scientific approach to the problem of change. In the context of the training program, we called this the "expected-to-observed strategy," and the trainees formalized it in a weekly meeting they called "group sharing of self-study." The strategy is basically a simple one: a problem exists; a course of action and a rationale for taking the action are proposed; a prediction of expected outcome is made; results are observed; and a revised strategy is set in motion if necessary. We tried to make this over-all strategy explicit in discussing methods for change and in relation to the trainees' role development and their relationships with other people. It was the core of what we tried to get at through the research-methods study group.

Stating expecteds about oneself and the program was a part of self-study sessions during Phase 1, but both trainees and staff found it a frustrating and often pointless experience. The trainees complained of a lack of structure. During Phase 2 they developed a specific outline for formulating expecteds. They were to state, in writing, a problem they had in work or personal relationships; to propose a way to handle the problem; to give a rationale for the proposed action; and to predict its result. The proposed action and the prediction were to be phrased clearly and concretely enough for the other trainees to observe whether or not the action and the result actually came about. The expecteds were presented to the group, and observations of how the actions had turned out were discussed by both the trainees and their peers two or three weeks later.

This structure was designed by the older trainees and accepted with some grumbling by the new ones. The problem now seemed to lie in the nature of the expecteds that the participants formulated. They sometimes had a moralistic quality ("I will try to talk less and listen to others more") or were vague in tone and intent ("I will work harder on writing"), despite efforts to state the goals in observable ways. It never seemed really clear to the trainees as a whole why they were engaged in this activity, despite continued efforts to relate the strategy to the work of program-development assistants. Some resented putting themselves on display and being made responsible to the group.

In Phase 3, the trainees decided to focus this activity on task achievement and to reserve personal development for the living-learning groups. Most of the expecteds now concerned the amount of work to be completed in a given time, and stressed the time of day during which the trainee was to be observed at a particular task. Predictions still tended to be unrealistic; but in evaluating the activity at the end of the project, the trainees felt it had helped push them toward accomplishment and organization of their efforts. Thus, though attention was not given to the problems that made it hard to get work done on time, the result was some change in actual behavior.

This activity was concerned with the trainees' own development, but the point of view it represented permeated other project activities. How does one plan for change in a systematic way? How are hypotheses formulated, and how are they revised in the face of evidence that sheds light on their plausibility? How can one differentiate between program planning based on an inner certainty (one "knows" the right thing to do) and programs based upon statable hypotheses that allow both the collection of evidence and program modification in the face of evidence? This kind of a stance toward social action is difficult for many people (including many social-science graduate students) to live with, but we submit it as one contribution psychologists can make, along with professionals from other disciplines, in approaching community problems.

Differences among Trainees

The project provides evidence, if further evidence is needed, that there is considerable unused potential for productive work on the part of persons the community has rejected. It leaves untouched the question of how widespread this potential is and under what conditions it can best be realized.

Our present formulations are crude. Our experiences suggest that a mixture of inner strength, specific training, personal supports, and environmental opportunity is necessary, that this mix varies with the individual and probably also with the environmental setting and task to be performed.

We have no measure of the extent to which each trainee developed understanding of either the content or the philosophy of the training program. We would judge that such understanding varied widely over the 18 trainees and that the variation has had little to do with later performance. Apparently, both efforts at self-aggrandizement and efforts to "get with" a cause can motivate toward success.

As a matter of data, the trainees who got into difficulty were all Caucasian. Only four of the ten Caucasian trainees are still in program-development work, while all eight of the minority-group trainees are working successfully. For the former group—those with greater initial access to the opportunity structure—personal hang-ups appear to have been more contributory to their getting into trouble in the first place and continue to plague their postprogram behavior. On the other hand, it is also true that in the fields in which the trainees are now working it has become a distinct advantage to be black. We are having difficulty in making an appropriate job referral for a Caucasian trainee who wants to return to program-development work.

There appears to be a tremendous drive on the part of many of the trainees to become a part of the Establishment. Our initial conception of having the trainees serve as linkers with others like themselves was quickly shattered. The trainees have done extremely well in relating to middle-management agency personnel. Few have been interested in identifying themselves with the downtrodden. These role shifts occurred very rapidly.

The amount and kind of personal support needed by the trainees, both off and on the job, have varied widely. Some seem born to negotiate any system, including a social-agency one, once they are given access to it. Others have never found a comfortable role, or have been comfortable only in certain types of employment situations. The trainees have differed also in their dependence on project staff for personal or financial support, in their ability to utilize their peers effectively for such support, and in their ability to form supportive relationships on their own.

Participation and Peer Involvement

It is commonplace to say that people should have a say in determining their own destiny. It is surprisingly hard to put this into practice, unless the professional pulls out completely. The battles with staff during the first training phase—polarized around the question "How do we know we can trust you?"—made almost any kind of goal-directed effort impossible. Staff were continually pushed into a position of "You tell us what to do," from which they were then attacked for doing so. The trainees, it was clear, often had no idea of what staff were talking about, and were extremely touchy about admitting it. The only part of the program that escaped criticism was the seminar on social issues in which the trainee teams took turns preparing papers on a self-selected topic and delivering the papers to the other trainees and staff. This was also the one learning activity in which staff had no role.

The problem was how to involve the trainees maximally in planning and carrying out the program when they approached the training situation from a position of ignorance, how to avoid an authority-learner relationship when the trainees brought little relevant knowledge and experience. What we hoped to provide was a statement of goals and a philosophy about personal development, giving the trainees maximum opportunity to plan ways in which the goals would be reached.

The training program did not actually take hold until the second phase, and its relative success during that phase is probably due chiefly to the unplanned contingency of having three of the eight Phase 1 trainees denied parole. These three spent the next four months writing a detailed history and critique of the Phase 1 program and plans for Phase 2 training, all with minimum consultation with staff. The Phase 2 program was both more ambitious and more structured than staff had or would have planned. For example, instead of a two-week orientation, with visits by institution and department staff and outside consultants, the trainees were shown the location of the dining hall, then told to go out and conduct a survey. The trainees also took over responsibility for all training functions from the outset, using the "olders" as consultants.

As a group, the Phase 2 and 3 trainees worked harder than those in Phase 1. There were no longer complaints of "I don't know what to do," but of "You're jamming the system," and these plaints were now directed to peers, not staff. It was not that the older trainees were always more skilled at evoking participation—they too could easily take on an authority-expert role—but that their involvement and expertise gave an accessible role model, a demonstration of staff faith in trainee potential, a more visible account of failure to meet expectations, and an opportunity to argue or disagree without fear of losing face. Moreover, it broke up the staff-inmate game many of the men were used to playing.

Because of the demands of the field program, available staff time was cut in half for Phase 2. By Phase 3, staff was almost nonexistent. In terms of present performance, there is no demonstrable difference between the functioning of the trainees in the three groups.

Trainee Development

Because the trainees were so dispersed and so mobile geographically, a consistent field training program was impossible. The project director tried to meet regularly with small groups of trainees around job problems, but this proved difficult to carry out consistently. During Phase 2, there were several meetings of trainees working in the field and in the institution, out of which came the job of project coordinator, a trainee whose function was to troubleshoot with job and personal problems, to write a project newsletter, and to keep the trainees and staff in touch with one another. As project funds ran out, this activity had to stop. At this time the trainees are in reasonably close touch with one another, despite being scattered in jobs across the country, and most are still in touch with the original project staff.

As expected, performance has varied among the trainees. Some have done consistently well; some have performed unevenly; most have shown steady growth in skill and in assurance. As a group, they have acquired some impressive skills. They can develop and write proposals; they can plan and administer manpower training programs; they can write job descriptions and plan career sequences; they can negotiate with civil-service, employment, and education systems; they can provide technical consultation to social agencies. When they left the training program, these skills were rudimentary, but they were skills not usually found at all in graduate students or in the staffs of most social agencies. In the years since, the skills have become considerable.

On most jobs, the trainees worked with a minimum of supervision. Many moved quickly into positions of substantial responsibility, often responsibility for which the project gave them little or no preparation. Some became anxious and left, others assumed the responsibility eagerly. Most of the trainees did well when the job was fairly structured, but some found problems when structure and close supervision were lacking. In the beginning the trainees did better on short-term, high-involvement projects with a clearly visible goal—they were impressive in their capacity to work to meet a crisis or a deadline. In this, they were probably not much different from other workers, but their ways of handling routine, monotony, and boredom were more likely to get them into trouble. They took on commitments quickly and enthusiastically, with little regard for their capacity to produce, and especially to produce within a stated time. When the deadline caught up with them, they sometimes handled it by walking away. Some let other interests—drinking, gambling, partying—take priority over showing up on the job. This kind of behavior has lessened markedly over time, especially as the trainees have gained confidence in and reward for their developing skills.

Employers were generally enthusiastic on their early contacts with the trainees. However, the trainees did not always wear well, and several of the employers became very unhappy about erratic job behavior, particularly carelessness about showing up on time or explaining absences. When the situation became too tense—and it sometimes did—the project hired the trainee and tried to work with him. There was in the early months a great deal of tolerance for sloppy behavior, and this tolerance has on the whole paid off.

In general, the trainees still in program-development work have been the most stable and the most independent in their job behavior. Those no longer working in this area have required the most support, from project staff and from employers. Some of these might still be in program development had more support been available.

Conclusion

Though our data are very limited, they are very encouraging about the potential within the rejects of the community. People not prepared for it by either education or experience can relatively easily "get with change" and with systematic study of change, and they can do this without being "cured." At the beginning, all the trainees wanted to rehabilitate young delinquents. Now they are excited about the possibilities of changing systems.

There is a great deal of changing to do. Few people are organized or prepared for it, including professionals. This study at least supports the position that there are significant sources of nonprofessional manpower in the community which can be developed to work effectively to bring about change in the community.

RELATED READINGS

Grant, J. D. The psychologist as an agent for scientific approaches to social change. In L. Abt (Ed.), *Progress in clinical psychology.* New York: Grune and Stratton, 1968.

Grant, J. D. Vital components of a model program using the offender in the administration of justice. In *Offenders as a correctional manpower resource.* Washington, D.C., Joint Commission on Correctional Manpower and Training, 1968.

Grant, J. D., & Grant, Joan. Staff and client participation: a new approach to correctional research. *Nebraska Law Rev.,* 1966, **45,** 702-716.

Pearl, A., & Riessman, F. *New careers for the poor.* New York: Free Press, 1965.

Toch, H. The study of man: the convict as researcher. *Trans-action,* 1967, **4,** 72-75.

IV

ISSUES AND
TRENDS IN EDUCATION
AND TRAINING

The final part of this volume concerns itself with the implications of the preceding parts and of developments in community psychology and community mental health in general, for the preparation of psychologists for work in the field. The four chapters focus on graduate education, on internship training at the postdoctoral level, and on the preparation of psychologists for research and consultation responsibilities.

Lipton and Klein, authors of Chapter 15, developed one of the pioneering university-based programs for education in community psychology. Their chapter characterizes their orientation to community psychology as the study and understanding of man in his habitat. They endeavor to develop in students not only a knowledge of community but also a sense of community, and their curriculum focuses on a spectrum of skills for relating to the community and on a conceptual framework with which to integrate these components. They describe the different perspectives brought by their students from clinical, counseling, personality, and social psychology. Their thoughtful appraisals of the pedagogical challenges they have encountered should be sources of stimulation for those psychology departments now developing analogous programs.

The Boston conference participants underscored the need for the development of internship programs as well as for graduate education. In Chapter 16, Kalis describes one program which is oriented to the preparation of clinicians for indirect, in contrast to direct, community-service roles. Her chapter gives a flavor of the variety and complexity of the community experience which works toward the simultaneous development of a number of intervention skills. Like Lipton and Klein, she emphasizes the need for appropriate role models, stressing the contributions of psychological knowledge in a necessarily interdisciplinary field. She gives attention to the modifications of orientation and technique relevant for clinicians entering the community and suggests that a multidisciplinary program can help to delineate the unique, as well as the generic, contributions of each profession.

Baler, in Chapter 17, articulates the urgent need for basic and applied research, addressing himself to the preparation of psychologists as community mental-health research specialists. He develops the thesis that the task of graduate education in this regard consists in the development of basic trust, feelings of competence, and a sense of identity. And he suggests that much of this development can begin at the undergraduate level and proceed stepwise throughout a student's total preparation for scientific and professional functioning.

Baler's implicit plea that psychology as a whole reorient itself to meaningful problems is echoed at the community level by Libo, both in his chapter on preparing psychologists for multiple functions in community consultation and in his addendum reminder that "Tourism is not enough." Just as the Boston conferees designated community psychology as the emerging new field and community mental health as a subdivision thereof, Libo indicates that while he is focusing on the training of psychologists, he feels that his recommendations should be applicable to the other mental-health disciplines as well.

This multidisciplinary emphasis on the nature of the field, the knowledge base, and the forms of training underlie the concern of all the authors, not only with the unique contributions of psychologists but also with what psychologists need to learn from other disciplines and with the generic aspects of community mental-health research and practice which cut across disciplinary boundaries. Thus, while Part IV, on education and training, might be expected to focus almost exclusively on the preparation of psychologists, like the remainder of the volume the concerns of the authors hopefully should generalize to other professions as well.

CHAPTER 15

Training Psychologists for Practice and Research in Problems of Change in the Community

Herbert Lipton and Donald C. Klein

For several years now, the authors have been conducting a training program in community psychology, under the auspices of the National Institute of Mental Health, that deals with practice and research in problems of change.[1] This program is intended to train clinical, counseling, and social and personality graduate students in psychology to study and to intervene in community groups and institutions. The program is sponsored jointly by the psychology department of Boston University and the Human Relations Center, a university-wide facility at Boston University which aims to stimulate instruction, research, and community services in applied behavioral science in all schools and departments.

The purpose of this paper is to describe, first, the orientation we have taken to community psychology; second, the goals and content of the training program; and third, some of the major issues and problems we have encountered.

THE ORIENTATION OF THE TRAINING PROGRAM

For us, "community psychology" refers as much to an orientation to the study of human behavior as it does to an area of knowledge or a set of professional practices. This orientation is to the study and understanding of man in his habitat. Community psychology therefore is concerned with the reciprocal relation of individuals and their environments, and with the development of ways in which interventions designed to foster more adequate

[1]The training program described in this chapter is supported by USPHS Training Grant No. MH 10226, from the National Institute of Mental Health.

person-environment relationships can best be effected. The purpose of our training program is to contribute to knowledge and understanding of these matters and thus to help map the significant features and boundaries of the terrain that is community psychology.

THE GOALS AND CONTENT OF THE PROGRAM

Deriving from this general orientation, we see our training program serving at least three major instructional goals. The first of these goals is to develop in the psychologist a greater awareness of and responsiveness to important community needs, to develop a "sense of community," as well as an appreciation of the community as a functional system. The second is to enable the psychologist to experiment with, and to learn and develop, professional and scientific skills which can be tested and then usefully applied in the community. The third is to develop a conceptual framework which would serve to integrate the first two program goals.

Let us examine in more detail how we implemented our program during its first three years, the kinds of backgrounds the students brought to the program, and some of the problems and learnings we experienced. As already mentioned, the program in community psychology is intended to train students in clinical, counseling, and social and personality psychology. It is geared for advanced students, and provides now a total of eight stipends at the third- or fourth-year level (in the first two years six stipends were available). An option for a second year in the program is possible. Sixteen different students, equally divided between the clinical and counseling programs and the social and personality program, have participated in Community Psychology Training in its first three years of operation. The program is conducted largely in the Human Relations Center, and there is embedded within a multidisciplinary fellowship program.

The program consisted of three major components: formal course work, field placements, informal discussion and reading. In addition to courses taken in the specialty, each student was required to take both a one-semester practicum, which was devoted to the development of sensitivity, diagnostic acumen, and behavioral skills in helping others in the process of collaborative change, and a one-semester proseminar devoted to the theory and principles of community and organizational change. Additional courses offered at the Human Relations Center were recommended and were taken by the students as appropriate. These included a seminar on psychological consultation, a seminar on evaluation research, an advanced practicum in human relations, as well as either the basic or advanced two-week residential summer workshop in human relations. Two new offerings were available to students last year. One was a graduate seminar on community psychology, in which a psychological understanding of community processes and the role of the psychologist in the community as researcher, consultant, practitioner, and planner were studied. The other was a two-week summer residential laboratory in community relations and community development, in which intergroup problems in the community were studied through a combination of experiential techniques and seminars. Courses in other departments of the university were also available; for example, courses in the epidemiological approach to the study of mental illness and in community conflict and change. Faculty consisted of members of the psychology department, staff of the Human Relations Center, as well as an adjunct faculty drawn from members of other departments of the university and specialists from outside the university, in psychology and in other related fields.

An informal community-psychology discussion group was organized, holding weekly meetings, for the purpose of helping to form a group identification for the individual students as well as to integrate course work, field work, and other experiences. In these discussions, the outlines of a conceptual framework for thinking about community problems were also being developed. This discussion group generated the following kinds of activities: arranged for brief field visits by groups of students to representative facilities in the areas of community mental health, community-development and antipoverty programs, intergroup relations, and educational systems; arranged for talks by faculty and community specialists in these areas; discussed these areas together as well as undertook relevant reading; worked on a definition of the field of community psychology through discussion and through the writing of papers on the subject at the beginning and the end of the year; participated in special training events such as a community-simulation exercise; and participated in a group study of the counseling needs of students at the university.

Field placements were established for each student, suited as much as possible to the individual's interests and needs, in order to provide direct experience with community problems and with the beginning development of the repertoire of professional and scientific skills required to participate in developing approaches to these problems. The field placements varied in time from 1½ to 4 days a week, depending on the individual student's level of training. They included activities that in some cases were external to the university, in other cases joint undertakings of the community and the university, and in still other cases primarily sponsored by the university. Some representative activities and their settings included: organization of a research program for the state Commission Against Discrimination; development of a preprogram interview of participants, and analysis of interviews for a workshop on the development of metropolitan leadership; participant-observation, social action, and interagency planning experience in an urban neighborhood house; individual assessment experience, consultation on groups, and cross-institutional analysis of approaches to the management of geriatric problems; experience in multilevel consultation and counseling with a voluntary self-help organization and with urban school systems; development of a proposal and early planning of a program to introduce human-relations training in a suburban high-school setting where the school administration sought to reduce intergroup tensions and conflict; and service as an administrative intern in the department of mental health.

In addition to this basic framework of training and experience, students in the program received both formal and informal supervision in their field placements, gained knowledge of the roles and values of other disciplines through their interaction with Human Relations Fellows at the Center from several other fields (sociology, nursing, theology, business, philosophy, education) in courses and informally; and gained acquaintance with various other Center projects and research studies through discussion or active participation with staff.

AN EVALUATION OF THE PROGRAM

An evaluation of the program, arrived at in collaboration with the students and through an independent assessment made by members of the adjunct faculty, suggested several points we could take satisfaction from and several issues that will continue to challenge us. On the positive side, we were impressed with the sensitivity that the students developed to community needs and processes, the "sense of community" that was a first goal of our program. They developed a fine awareness of the urgent and continuing problems to which the psychologist has been responding and will be asked to respond in the areas of community mental health, education and retraining, intergroup relations, and community development. They became highly aware of the ubiquity of intergroup tensions and conflict taken in the largest sense, and of a prominent special case of this phenomenon which exists in the widespread isolation that has developed between social agencies. They became highly concerned over the general lack of preprogram planning for social services, including the assessment of needs, the definition of target population, and the feasibility of delivering services. And they responded to many other issues including: the conflict between central planners and potential recipients of services due to the lack of collaborative involvement of the latter; the problems of group formation; the multiple problems of consultation including the essential two-way nature of such a helping relationship; the reciprocal relation that exists between a person's or a group's feelings of lack of significance and involvement and the social structure or opportunity required to make possible feelings of significance; and the problems inherent in doing effective evaluation research, both methodological and inherent in the social reality.

We are now in a position to discuss the second goal of our program, the development of the professional and scientific skills that the community psychologist should have in order to function effectively in that setting. While admittedly generalizing from a small sample, we believe we have seen major differences in orientation, interest, and skill that students from the three specialties brought to our program. These differences, moreover, represent unique contributions that these specialties can make to practice and study in community psychology. The student from social psychology brings a knowledge of small groups and communication problems, familiarity with the concept of role, techniques for studying group dynamics, an interest in evaluation research, and a conceptual-theoretical orientation that makes him comfortable in dealing with large masses of data. However, he may not be as well prepared to move from the level of thought to the level of action and involvement.

The clinical student brings interests in motivation, personality organization, behavioral skewing and deviancy, and skills for inducing relearning, growth planning, decision making, and confrontation of conflict, on the individual and interpersonal levels. In contrast to the student from social psychology, he is more apt to intervene, to take action, to become involved with individuals and groups, to learn from the experience rather than from the collection of research data, and concomitantly, to be slower in moving from the realm of direct interpersonal experience to the realm of conceptualization.

The counseling student brings many of the interests and skills of the clinical student; in addition, he is perhaps more oriented to the reality of institutional and organizational life, and is more directed to the manipulation of this reality in his client's behalf. He, like the clinical student, seems to derive more satisfaction from intervention than from statistical or conceptual closure.

The preference toward action involvement or toward research which students seem to have during their first year in the program appears to be obviated for those students (and this is the majority) who stay in the program for two years. They seem more comfortable the second year in gaining experience with the other mode.

The emphasis throughout our program was to fit the student's interests and skills to the community problems, while at the same time making possible an extension of his interests and skills. All students in the program were exposed, through course work and through field placement, to the basic repertoire of practice and research skills, and we were pleased with the increased effectiveness they showed in the use of diagnostic, consultative, and evaluation skills.

Training in practice included a variety of relevant and necessary skills, some or all of which a given community psychologist would require: the application of clinical and therapeutic competence in times of unusual stress; facility in using diagnostic and consultative approaches at a number of different levels of organization; and capacities for involvement in planning, training, and social action.

The third goal of the program, the development of a conceptual framework, we might fairly say we are still approaching. The ubiquitous theme we have already mentioned, that ran through so much of our experience, was the existence of intergroup tension. There appear to be strong, pervasive forces which virtually assure social distance and often conflict between groups which differ from one another in some respect, such as age, sex, occupation, socioeconomic status, or beliefs. We have used the term "social cleavage" in considering these problems. With this divisive theme in the community as a major focus for further inquiry, the study of complementary integrative mechanisms in the community becomes crucial, and the relation of individual behavior and effectiveness to these social contexts becomes of primary importance.

PROBLEMS ENCOUNTERED IN THE PROGRAM

Several problems were encountered early in the program. A major pedagogical challenge remains: How can we best integrate, in the program, learning through experience and learning on the conceptual level? This problem showed several sides. At times it was seen in an individual student's predilection for exploring the affective or interpersonal aspects of the learning situation in contrast to another student's desire to go ahead with the task and the concepts (the former position was dubbed "T-grouping it"). Or it was seen as a desire to separate action from research, or vice versa, reflecting the kind of general issue Chein (1966) has raised regarding what he calls the opposition between scientism and clinicalism. Or at times the tension was between basic research and evaluation research. While we have no panacea to suggest for this major problem, the nature of the Human Relations Center, offering as it does a multidisciplinary and a multimodel approach to community problems, will enable us to continue pedagogical experiments dealing with the vital issue of valid ways in which knowledge is built.

Another problem is the tendency of clinical and counseling students to view the community selectively in terms of pathology and, in fact, the tendency of students in social psychology at times to follow suit, since the clinically oriented ones are the experts in this area. There is an allied tendency for many psychologists to view social problems symptomatically and to seek remedies on this level, whereas the sociologist or the political scientist would conceptualize the problem and its solution differently. More recently, through a more extensive use of adjunct faculty from different disciplines, and because of the increasing exposure students are receiving in systems theory, both in the university and in field settings, there appears to be both a diminution in the pathological view of community and a more balanced search for sources of community resources and creative energies.

A third significant problem is the lack of adequate role models for the student in community psychology. In more general terms, it is a problem because the guidelines for appropriate actions and skills are not available. More specifically, supervision in field placements represents a problem because, with the exception of the field of community mental health, there are few psychologists available to undertake the direct supervision of the student seeking a community-psychology experience. Apparently, few psychologists have made their way into fields of application like intergroup relations and community development. In the past year the number of psychologists in the community and the diversity of roles they play seem to have increased; however, this increase is found largely in the area of community mental health, followed by a small increase in the area of education. Consequently, we found ourselves serving dual roles: responsible for academic training on the one hand, and undertaking supervisory responsibilities for field placement on the other. From this vantage point, the need and appropriateness of training programs in community psychology are highlighted, in order that the penetration of psychologists into crucial problem areas in the community can occur.

REFERENCE

Chein, I. Some sources of divisiveness among psychologists. *Amer. Psychologist*, 1966, **21**, 333-342.

CHAPTER 16

Immersion in Community as a Training Approach: The Multiagency, Multimethod Field-Work Experience

Betty L. Kalis

Contributions to community psychology are being made by psychologists with many types of background, training, and experience. Concepts, methodology, research and action programs, all are developing and changing rapidly in this new and embryonic field. In some respects it may seem premature to design and implement training programs in a specialty which is shifting and for which the literature is still largely unwritten or subject to publication lags which render it outdated by the time it appears. But community mental-health practice, as an aspect of community psychology, demands approaches and skills not taught in traditional settings. Consequently, special academic and field-work programs are emerging in many parts of the country. This paper will describe certain features of the Langley Porter Community Mental Health Training Program,[1] an internship experience available for psychologists, as one model for field training. The chapter will then use this program description as a springboard for the discussion of selected training issues.

[1]The Langley Porter Community Mental Health Training Program, California Department of Mental Hygiene, is under the direction of M. Robert Harris, M.D. The full-time staff, in addition to the author, includes Joan Ablon, Ph.D., urban anthropologist; Rosalie M. Jones, R.N., M.S., mental-health nurse-consultant; Lida Schneider, A.M., A.C.S.W., social-work consultant. Part-time staff members are W. Reed Brockbank, M.D., and Lawrence Lurie, M.D., psychiatric consultants. Egon Bittner, Ph.D., formerly part-time sociologist in the program, made significant contributions to the program developments described in this paper. The views expressed in this chapter are those of the author and not the official position of the Department of Mental Hygiene.

THE MULTIDISCIPLINARY LANGLEY PORTER PROGRAM

The history and format of basic training in the Langley Porter program has been described by Harris, Kalis, and Schneider (1967). Although the program is based in a psychiatric institute and is under psychiatric direction, it has from the beginning been multidisciplinary with respect to both staff and trainees. Even its designation as "community mental health" rather than "community psychiatry" reflects the breadth of its conceptualization and its operation, the focus being on what the "mental-health professional" can bring to and learn from the community. The concept of "mental-health professional" refers to the clinically trained specialist, and the program was designed, and is therefore most appropriate, for the supplemental community training of clinicians. There may be aspects of the program which would be equally germane to the preparation of psychologists from other backgrounds, but discussion of training issues will center on the differences between community approaches and traditional clinical practice. Admission to the program is currently limited for psychologists to those who have completed clinical doctorates including a predoctoral internship. The advanced curriculum is a one- or two-year postdoctoral internship in the new specialty of community mental health.

The training experience is community-based, with institutional backup of seminars and supervision, as distinguished from those academically based programs which may have a field component to illustrate classroom principles. The postdoctoral psychology fellow is, in a very real sense, immersed in the community and emerges to stand back from his experience and conceptualize its relevance to him as a community psychologist. Thus, the role of participant-conceptualizer is from the outset a part of the internship.

THE FELLOW AND HIS NEIGHBORHOOD

Each fellow has a neighborhood of the city, designated as his geographic focus, with which to familiarize himself. He has no structured function in relation to the neighborhood and goes there uninvited—a far cry from both the assigned role of therapist and

the patient who seeks him out. The urban neighborhoods are selected on the basis of having some identifiable social-psychological
problems and, in San Francisco, invariably some clear ethnic characteristics. Usually, there is some form of community organization
devoted to neighborhood concerns, ranging from a neighborhood
association to an antipoverty council or a coalition devoted to
opposing redevelopment.

The fellow is encouraged to explore the neighborhood, to get to
know the people, the houses, the streets, the shops, and the transportation. He eats in its restaurants and makes small purchases in
a corner store, chatting with the shopkeepers. He assesses the
strengths, as well as the problems, of the area. He begins gradually,
through many channels, to get to know the wide variety of non-
mental-health professionals who work to maintain and improve
the functioning of the neighborhood and its inhabitants. For many
trainees, this is the first explicitly professional meeting with caretakers outside the mental-health field; and for many of the latter,
it is their first contact with mental-health workers, at least in non-
traditional guise.

At the same time, the fellow begins acquainting himself with
both Establishment and New Look resources and institutions in
the neighborhood. Community organization becomes something
more than a vague theoretical concept conjuring up images of
power structure, planning councils, boards, and committees (although for many psychologists even these classic images are new).
As a participant-observer, he learns first-hand about some of the
ethnic and social-class differences which comprise the texture of
community life. Much of his clinical experience has been with the
white middle class and its aspirants, and most trainees are unpre-
pared both for the modes of adaptation and the modes of communication they encounter in the broader community.

The goal in learning about a *specific* community is to find out
how to learn about *any* community. The field methods are familiar
ones to social scientists but by and large unfamiliar, and at least
initially uncomfortable, to the clinician. He brings with him, however, his background in individual and group dynamics and his
sensitivity to the nuances of verbal and nonverbal communication.
His interest in the motivational component of behavior and his
(hopefully) nonjudgmental stance can make him a fascinated lis-
tener in a new arena, but here, painfully, he must learn that com-

munication is two-way, that he cannot only listen but must give of himself as well.

The organizational triumvirate of health, education, and welfare services provides a useful template for the beginning understanding of community resources. To these three, however, must be added the administration of justice, for the neighborhood patrol cars and juvenile detail are crucial barometers of a facet of community functioning as well as an Establishment response to the neighborhood.

The fellow's introduction to the health department begins at the district health center, where he often finds that the health officer is exquisitely familiar with the demographic characteristics of the neighborhood and population approaches to prevention and services. He begins to translate these into terms which have import for psychological services. He sees mothers bringing their children to the child-health conferences and watches them interact with each other and with the pediatricians and nurses. Health education springs into action around innoculations and childbirth-preparation classes. He goes on home visits with the nurses and gets a new glimpse of how families in his neighborhood function and what their homes are like. He learns that nursing visits around growing families are family-oriented, not illness-oriented, and aspects of "prevention" and "focused intervention" take on new meaning.

In some areas, as in any urban complex, he finds that large numbers of elderly people are living alone, with no one to call on for such essentials as meals if they become home-bound. He watches the development of self-help programs that serve the broad needs of the whole group for relatedness and meaning in their lives as well as the specific needs of the disabled.

His first visit to the schools in his neighborhood may also be with the public-health nurse who serves them, but others will originate in the educational system. He meets principals, teachers, guidance and attendance workers, not in what may have been a previous role in a conference about a child with emotional difficulties, but to view the school as a basic institution with a community-serving and growth-promoting function. His visits to classrooms provide a perspective on the emotional climate in which children of the neighborhood spend so many of their waking hours, and on the teachers as prime community caretakers. He listens to the school board wrestle with problems of racial imbalance, nonachievers, and educationally handicapped, as the board tries to mediate the wishes of diverse but vocal community residents.

With the welfare worker, too, he visits homes of families receiving various categorical aids and struggling with multiple burdens of poverty, unemployment, illness, and despair. Back in the welfare-department office, he learns that here, as well, the coordination of federal, state, and local funds in the development of meaningful services is a complex task and that it proceeds with little explicit cognizance of parallel planning by other networks. Later, he will become puzzledly aware, for example, that planning for comprehensive health services is virtually independent of planning for mental-health services, just as planning for mental-retardation services has frequently been split off from the concern with mental-health needs. He will ponder the conflicts between parochialism and the need for coordination, and between historical and fiscal isolation and new conceptualizations wherein patterns of generic human needs transcend guild boundaries.

Thus, the psychology fellow begins to learn about the community—its structure, its people, its resources—and the networks of communication and influence which connect, and the gaps which separate, these various components. Community organization, development, and change are experienced as ongoing processes and as the essential "basic science" of community psychology. But course work in this science has been the province of schools of social work, and many of the organizations he contacts are staffed by professional social workers, albeit professionals with quite different outlooks from the psychiatric social workers who were so familiar and congenial in clinical settings. Moreover, the field methods he has been encouraged to adopt, and the variables they bring into focus, relate more to anthropology and sociology than to psychology, and research concerns with epidemiology and biostatistics are foreign to the journals he has habitually read.

His professional identity, usually just barely formed when he enters the program, is questioned in all of its aspects, and he sees peers from psychiatry, social work, and nursing in this program or allied programs raising the same "Who am I?" and "What am I doing here?" kinds of questions. His major supervisor is from his own discipline and provides a new role model, but he is also expected to consult regularly with staff members from other disciplines as well. In his initial moving out into the neighborhood, these multidisciplinary supervisors are often more specifically knowledgeable than his psychology supervisor.

He learns that each program staff member carries liaison responsibilities for a number of organizations and agencies. There is ongoing evaluation of the learning opportunities afforded by each of these community outposts as well as negotiation and renegotiation of contracts for the indirect services which may be rendered by program participants, staff and trainees alike. For as he becomes acquainted with the neighborhood and with community-organization and -development methods, he also begins, simultaneously, to learn other community-mental-health methods. He may serve on boards and committees, design and conduct a program evaluation or a community-research project, participate in mental-health educational efforts, relate to program planning and administration issues and problems, and become a mental-health consultant.

The role of mental-health consultant is cathected eagerly because of its superficial similarity to clinical roles. The fellow has regular assignments to designated organizations with a contractual arrangement involving an ongoing time commitment. He meets individuals and groups with a broadly conceived mandate for helpful intervention and problem-solving activity in relation to the organization's work. He is there as a mental-health specialist. There the similarity ends, and the differences are manifold, but he must often learn this slowly and with difficulty. In time he understands the comment by Altrocchi and Eisdorfer (1970) that "the most appropriate attitude of the consultant and the consultant-in-training in a community is eagerness to learn from the community."

He is a participant in the Head Start Center, getting to know teachers and aides as, side by side, they all bend to pick up toys or bundle up homeward-bound youngsters against the rain. At a committee meeting, he encounters the agency director from another consultation. In a discussion over lunch, he hears about an important development which will affect the budget of yet another consultee group. When he is assigned a consultation, he learns about the neighborhood in which the agency or organization is located and the people it serves. He is interested not only in the history of the consultation contract but in the history of the agency itself. He identifies its board members and their backgrounds and other community involvements, or he studies public laws or codes or codes under which services function. The daily paper becomes as important a part of his preparation as are professional journals and books.

A SUBJECT FOCUS AND
A NEIGHBORHOOD FOCUS

Further structure to his immersion in the community is afforded by a subject focus of his own choosing in addition to the neighborhood focus. The two may or may not be interrelated, but his program-research effort is expected to be in this area. The subject focus may be broad or narrow, but the fellow explores its relationship to community mental health and acquaints himself with those individuals, groups, and organizations that are involved in planning and services in the subject area. One psychology fellow in the basic program was able to combine a neighborhood focus in Chinatown with a subject focus on immigration and acculturation in relation to mental health. In a detailed report, he commented:

In examining the extreme difficulty in "reaching" and in providing services to the Chinese community, although a variety of important factors such as the language problem are patent, the importance of a xenophobic factor is not to be discounted. Many Chinese, especially those who have lived for years with the fears of an illegal immigrant, will have nothing to do with any public body or agency even if it means starving as a result. Similar considerations arise also for new immigrants, who must wait five years before they can establish citizenship and are in the interim terrified of blotting their copy-books. This becomes especially important in respect to psychiatric problems since being without mental disorder is a condition of citizenship.

Immigrants are now arriving in San Francisco at the rate of some 5,000 a year and Chinatown is for them both a buffer zone of gentle adaptation and a fixation zone. The situation facing them in terms of housing and employment is critical and is becoming more so. For many the realities of Chinatown come as a great shock after the long years of glowing reports coming from friends and relatives on the "golden mountain." Though a number were better off in Hong Kong, hardly any return there, and the new immigrants, too, will write back glowing testimonials to Chinatown, San Francisco, since shame is intolerable. The new immigrant, unless he speaks English or has special skills, is confined to the saturated labor market in Chinatown and the relative who supports him initially will soon want him off his back. He is likely to be in debt to his sponsor for a long time to come.

... It is already clear that there are many sources of stress within the

Chinese community, particularly for the new immigrant, that might be expected to take their toll in mental health. Children, adults, and old people all have their own peculiar conflicts. Special factors ... include the frequent incidence of lengthy separations between family members resulting from restrictive immigration laws (often in combination with financial difficulties), the common practice of both parents working excessively long hours to make ends meet with its consequences for their children, and the special problems attending wives brought from Hong Kong following arranged marriages (a declining but continuing practice). Actual assessment of mental health in the community is a difficult matter owing to the inadequacy of treatment facilities, the traditional Chinese view of "mental" problems, and the reluctance of the Chinese to avail themselves of services (John H. Davis, Ph.D., unpublished manuscript).

The paper from which this quotation was excerpted was part of this fellow's seminar report on his subject focus. The seminar component of the advanced program is an important feature of the internship experience. For the first six months he is expected to attend the twice-weekly basic seminars (if he has not been in the basic program), which include discussions of principles and methods, introduction to a number of community resource people, and reviews of field experiences. Suggested readings are provided for each seminar topic, and the advanced fellows use the bibliographies from these references as one source for uncovering additional pertinent literature.

FORMAL LEARNING EXPERIENCES

In addition, the weekly advanced colloquium is a forum for discussion of developing conceptualization in the field of community mental health and for interaction with program staff as well as with invited institute staff who are involved and interested in community work. As the year proceeds, the fellows assume planning responsibility for the colloquium, including the responsibility for presenting to the group aspects of their own work in the field.

An unusual additional formal learning opportunity began in 1967 and will continue throughout 1970. The department of psychiatry and the program director, together with the psychiatry department and director from the University of Louisville, are hosts to 15 psychiatric educators with training responsibilities in community mental health. Two-week workshops are held twice-yearly around core topics in the field, with invited participants from around the country; program staff and fellows attend these sessions as well.

The supervisory-tutorial conferences, however, are probably the richest institute-based learning experience for staff and fellows alike. Here, issues of role diffusion and differentiation can be explored, concepts of preventive intervention refined, crisis theory developed, and ecological hypotheses shaped. Questions of technique can be examined in relation to yesterday's field experience; philosophy and changing professional ethics can be debated, and frustrations and satisfactions shared and exchanged.

SOME TRAINING ISSUES ENCOUNTERED

As this program, which has involved to date about 20 psychologists in addition to many trainees from other disciplines, has developed, a number of training issues have arisen. It has become clear that effective functioning in the field of community mental health requires more than the extension of activities outside the institution and the addition of indirect services to one's armamentarium. For the clinician, several major shifts in focus are required, and the goals of preparation should include the facilitation of these shifts. The phrase "shift in focus" reflects the philosophy that clinical training and experience are relevant and not to be abandoned but that they serve as a foundation on which other perspectives are built.

The psychologist in particular brings to such a program not only a research degree and a knowledge of methodology and statistics, but the inquiring stance which underlies this knowledge and is so vital in a field whose parameters are still in the process of definition, whose methods are in the infancy of development, and whose data are rich but unmined. The psychologist brings also a background in the area of normal development, particularly child development, and a basic grounding in the psychology of adaptation or ego psychology, not just an exclusive exposure to psychopathology. His knowledge of the latter and his knowledge of individual and group dynamics are important assets shared with clinicians from other backgrounds.

Clinical training and experience, with their emphasis on pathology, often obscure the background in normal development, and in our view the first shift in focus is from this exclusive concern with psychopathology to an emphasis on adaptation and functioning. The community psychologist must become somewhat less concerned with what impedes and immobilizes and more involved with those factors which facilitate and maintain coping and adaptation. While it is a truism that comprehensive assessment must involve both adaptive and maladaptive components of a situation, both the assessment and the interpretation of growth-promoting factors are difficult for clinically trained professionals to attend to in their early work in the community.

One example that helps elucidate this point is that a significant finding for community mental health is inherent in the Midtown Manhattan Study (Srole et al., 1962), but seldom commented on. Of the Home Survey Sample, 58 per cent were described as either mildly or moderately impaired psychiatrically, and this figure is often cited as reflecting the need for additional mental-health services. The equally fascinating implication, however, derives from the fact that these categories describe people who "present significant signs of emotional disturbance *without apparent constriction or disability in discharging the ordinary functions or roles of adult life*" (Srole et al., 1962, p. 135; emphasis added). A vital challenge for the community psychologist is to determine how these people continue to function.

The emphasis upon adaptation requires a broadening of the concept of responsibility from the mental-health professional as the helper of choice to a large number of other professionals and nonprofessionals, and perhaps most importantly the involvement of individuals, families, and groups in the planning for their own needs and the resolution of their own difficulties. Teamwork with teachers, general physicians, probation officers, and employment counselors is often easier to achieve than giving ghetto residents more than a token voice on the board of a center that is to serve their neighborhood or including patients and their families in treatment-planning conferences.

The community psychologist must also move from consideration of the individual as the inevitable center of the social system, with family and school and job viewed only as they relate to him, to a flexible approach in which the social-system center varies according to the subject of study, and wherein the over-all social matrix is continually the ground on which figures are imposed. Thus, a community psychologist relating to a program for unwed teenage mothers may need to be aware simultaneously of: the client who is struggling with the decision of keeping her child or relinquishing it; the putative father who is weighing the prognosis for marriage against the kinds of responsibilities he can assume without marriage; the teacher searching for relevant classroom materials at a time when her pupils' need-hierarchies are loaded with their pregnancy concerns; the social worker who is valiantly striving to coordinate widely disparate community resources to meet the mothers' multiple needs; the family-planning specialist who is searching for ways to provide information *before* pregnancy occurs; and so on. While all of these participants in this particular human drama are responding to a common *event*, the pregnancy, their definition of the issue and alternative possibilities for its resolution must appropriately differ for each. The psychologist, then, must be able to move flexibly in relation to these different points of view, and with as clear as possible a notion of the population at risk, the various levels of prevention inherent in each potential approach, and above all the relevance of the social issue to the mental health of the mothers and their babies.

The need for an awareness of the total social matrix and an approach which centers successively on various social systems requires a concomitant shift wherein intrapsychic variables assume a subordinate role to ecological considerations. While the ecological viewpoint emphasizes the *interaction* between intraorganismic and environmental variables, many clinicians new to community mental health tend to conceptualize the work as abandoning intrapsychic considerations, attending only to external forces, and intervening solely as an environmental manipulator or social engineer. Just as they may have previously erred in discounting the importance of social, economic, ethnic, and political factors as they contribute to the understanding of behavior, so in their new enthusiasm they may give these factors exclusive importance and fail to recognize the relevance of individual dynamics or the ability of people to affect external components of their lives. The definition of ecological variables is the greatest conceptual challenge for community mental health. The delineation of interaction variables requires attention not only to the contribution of the ecology to the behavior of its members but to the members' influence in the changing ecological balance. It is here that the rapprochement between clinical psychology and the social sciences must occur, not through the former giving cognizance to environmental factors and the latter taking into account intrapsychic ones, but by their working together in a common arena toward new interactional conceptualizations.

While it is clear that psychology, like many other professions, has unique contributions to make to community mental health which require both educative and research efforts within the discipline, the need for many kinds of professionals to work and learn together is also obvious. The complex nature of the field will, as it develops, bring together many scientists and practitioners who have previously had little if any contact. They will learn from, and contribute to, each other and to the conceptualization and practice of community mental health. They will sort out the generic concerns of all who are attracted to so broadly defined an area from the more specific interests of various specialists. It is to meet this need for multidisciplinary study and collaboration that the Langley Porter Community Mental Health Training Program has been developed and is continually enriched. While certainly not to be regarded as *the* model for the preparation of psychologists, it is one approach with appropriateness and relevance at this stage in the development of the field.

REFERENCES

Altrocchi, J., & Eisdorfer, C. Apprentice-collaborator field training in community psychology: the Halifax County program. In I. Iscoe & C. D. Spielberger (Eds.), *Community psychology: perspectives in training and research.* New York: Appleton-Century-Crofts, 1970.

Harris, M. R., Kalis, Betty L., & Schneider, Lida. Training for community mental health in an urban setting. *Amer. J. Psychiat.*, 1967, **124** (Suppl.), 20-29.

Srole, L., Langner, T. S., Michael, S. T., Opler, M. K., Rennie, T. A. C. *Mental health in the metropolis: the midtown Manhattan study.* New York: McGraw-Hill, 1962.

CHAPTER 17

Training for Research in Community Mental Health

Lenin A. Baler

Concerning research in the community mental health field, there would appear to be consensus on two points. First, the most urgent need is for basic and applied research on a wide scale. This assertion occurs in epidemic frequency in most official documents, conference reports, position papers, and symposia. It also typically appears in more muted form in the last paragraph of agency annual reports. Second, among the various specialties in mental health, psychology is expected, by virtue of its constitutionally defined self-image as both a science and a profession, to be ethically committed to doing research. To be sure, the relative ratio of research to practice is sensibly permitted to vary with the interest intensity and competence level of the individual psychologist, but university training programs have always operated on the assumption that the individual psychologist's direct and indirect contribution to research should be well above zero.

Now, if the community at large can confront the mental health professions with the challenge of enabling legislation and logistical support to launch a "bold, new approach" to the prevention and control of mental disorders, it would seem only fitting that psychologists accept the in-group challenge to train students so that they will be equipped with the requisite skills and motivation to

Reprinted with permission of the author and Behavioral Publications from *Community Mental Health Journal*, Vol. 3, No. 3 (Fall 1967), pp. 250-253. The article is a revision of "The Psychologist as Community Mental Health Research Specialist," a paper read at the Annual Meeting of the American Psychological Association, New York, 1966.

make a contribution to community mental health research that will indeed be well above zero.

Manpower resources are such that students at all levels of training ought to be of some value in the research effort. It is certainly regrettable that the large number of talented psychology students who do not go beyond the Bachelor's degree are lost to the manpower pool as potential research assistants and technicians frankly because their present undergraduate education has just about zero transfer value for community research tasks. Present doctoral training, in particular in clinical psychology, automatically produces, at least in the opinion of several observers, negative transfer value. Finally, staff members involved in postdoctoral community mental health specialist programs sometimes feel that it is too late and that as in psychotherapy few patients can really be "cured" in spite of best efforts!

The thesis of this paper is that training institutions need to socialize students early and continuously for the role of community mental health researcher.

One cannot, in fairness, identify a problem without proferring at least a few speculations as to the required remedy. Perhaps the simplest way of doing this is to organize the discussion around three concepts universally used when psychologists talk about the socialization process: basic trust, feelings of competence, and sense of identity.

BASIC TRUST

It is painful to note that psychologists who as professionals seek so earnestly to promote mental health in others by arguing the case for basic trust as nuclear to maturity in any social role have often failed to secure this "highest good" for themselves within their own training institutions. The reference here, of course, is to the long-endemic irrational and destructive clash between the so-called scientists and the practitioners within university psychology departments and between academic staff and community line workers. Probably few students, indeed, have failed to perceive this climate of distrust and consequently to suffer constraints upon their own full development as psychologists.

An articulate and thoroughly incisive analysis of this situation has recently been made by Chein (1966). He takes a close look at the problem as a social process, as the clash of two subcultures, and as a political conflict. One of the serious consequences of this basic distrust is the derogation of scholarship. In Chein's words, "blatant ignorance, stereotyping, and lack of comprehension become a sufficient basis for oracular pronouncements on the incompetence of the outermost out-group to make any significant contributions to psychology." Particularly disconcerting is that community mental health workers (whether in research or practice) currently constitute the most likely candidates for Chein's "outermost out-group" label.

The solution Chein proposes seems entirely reasonable. He says, "I am, thus, not pleading for a burial of differences. On the contrary, I am saying that we should open them up and bring them out from behind the fog of interpersonal and intergroup hostility. It is time for us to grow up and stop confusing our interpersonal and intergroup problems with the business of psychology." It needs only to be added that a similar solution is applicable to the divisiveness between psychologists and psychiatrists if they are to work really productively together in practice and research in the community mental health field.

If the present schism between the scientist and the practitioner continues unabated in the university, the university will remain a grossly inept socializing agent for training psychologists in community mental health. The academic scientist can produce much useful research even though he may escape into scientism. The clinical practitioner can contribute significantly to human welfare even though he may escape into clinicalism. In contrast, a line community mental health researcher cannot function with such a one-sided identity as scientist-practitioner (Gelfand & Kelly, 1960). This is so because there is no such thing as community research apart from community practice. As long as psychologists are reared in a climate of distrust that demands schizophrenic adjustments to the scientist and practitioner roles, competent community mental health researchers will remain in very short supply.

FEELINGS OF COMPETENCE

One normally prefers to do what he feels competent to do. Psychologists as presently trained are all too frequently dramatically incompetent to undertake community research. Even senior psychologists enrolled in postdoctoral community mental health training programs often lack rudimentary practical knowledge of community organization, are totally inexperienced in operating in the real community in regard to sanction problems or collaboration with nonprofessionals, and find embryonic their mastery of relevant technical research skills, such as questionnaire construction, survey methodology, and the art of just plain naturalistic observation. This situation is rather appalling when one recalls that in the first lecture in introductory psychology the instructor is apt to write on the board the universally accepted formula "Behavior results from the interaction between the person and his environment." It is hard to understand how the study of the environment (in terms of the customary goals of description, prediction, and control) is subsequently so neglected conceptually in the curriculum and neglected experientially in field assignments. As pointed out earlier, adequate socialization for the role of community mental health research worker must begin early and occur continuously.

Community Practicum

Absolutely mandatory is the development of a series of graded community practicum experiences that begin as early as possible in undergraduate training in psychology. These can vary from simple homework exercises, tutorial supervision, clerkship, and extra assignments to summer apprenticeship and internship placement. What can be the objections to this? It will "water down" the intellectual quality of college work? Nonsense. It has every chance of doing just the opposite by enriching the student's awareness of the nature of reliable and valid data, the utility of theories and conceptual models for formulating hypotheses, and the operational complexity of research designs required to test such hypotheses. Another objection may be that the average undergraduate is not mature enough to carry out and to benefit from such assignments. Again, nonsense; look at what young people are able to do and learn as mental health volunteers, as Vista workers in the poverty program, as "big brothers and sisters" in delinquency control. The main requirement for success is that the community practicum be overtly and honestly valued by the faculty and integrated thoroughly into the formal classroom subject matter. Basic trust thus continues to be of overriding importance.

What are some specific examples of practicum experiences of potential value in the early socialization of psychologists as community mental health research workers? Space permits a sketchy listing of only five:

1. For a given community, obtain the U.S. census data for 1950 and 1960. What demographic and socioeconomic changes have occurred? Discuss the implications in terms of the need for mental health services of different types.

2. Administer a questionnaire that taps attitudes toward mental illness of members of the local police force. Discuss the results with reference to the need for a mental health in-service training program for the police.

3. In collaboration with the staff of the local high school, compute the overall dropout rate over the past five years. See if the rate varies with some other variable, such as age or sex.

4. A certain health bill is coming up for legislative hearings. Attend these and observe what agencies present arguments pro and con. Follow up with individual interviews to ascertain agency goals and motivations behind the official position on the bill.

5. During the summer, volunteer to serve as an aide to a public health nurse. Accompany her on home visits. Keep a daily log and write a final report highlighting how her job involves mental health work directly and indirectly.

To summarize at this point, the contention here is that unless psychologists are socialized early in some fashion along the lines suggested above they will be unlikely to develop a serious interest in community mental health research during doctoral training or later in their career.

Formal Classroom Instruction

The acquisition of feelings of competence as a community research worker requires not only the community practicum experience just discussed but also is dependent upon adequate classroom instruction in relevant research logic and methodology. That something is very much amiss here has been recognized by many. Recently Marvin Dunnette (1966) has cleverly pinpointed the details of the problem. Taking his cue from Berne (1964), Dunnette examines the games that psychologists play in the name of science but which lead "down the primrose path to nonscience" and to nonsense. One instance of Dunnette's slashing insight can be seen in his definition of folderol as "those practices characterized by ... wasteful fiddle-faddle—including tendencies to be fixated on theories, methods, and points of view, conducting 'little' studies with great precision ... asking unimportant or irrelevant questions ... coining new names for old concepts. ..."

Learning how to "play games" has its own reward, to be sure. The reward clearly is not, however, feelings of competence in skills relevant to community mental health line research. A solution is exceedingly difficult to come by, because the acquired love of gamesmanship perpetuates itself as each new generation of students passes through the university. A moral injunction "Let's stop playing games!" merely raises the suspicion that some fascinating new game is about to be played.

A few psychologists have managed to reject the "establishment" and happily have been socialized in the real world of social commitment and social action research. Part of the solution to the problem under discussion is somehow to get these individuals to accept appointments on the faculties of our academic institutions. Another part of the solution lies in getting some of the more promising university scientists out of the ivory tower to function, not as mere alienated consultants, but as line researchers on the community team. Maybe then students can learn the basic research skills they really need: the ability to accept without paralyzing anxiety the fact that nonexperimental data is unwieldy, the ability to see a correlation based on naturalistic observation, not as an object of disparagement, but as a challenge to explore further whether the relationship is direct, indirect, or simply spurious, the ability to undertake applied research without feeling that one is committing an unforgivable sin.

SENSE OF IDENTITY

The task of completing the socialization of the psychologist for the role of community mental health research worker falls necessarily to the community mental health field agency itself. It is here "on the firing line" that the sense of identity must be firmed up and spelled out. It is here where the action is that community research problems can most realistically be formulated. It is here where the newcomer must learn to get along with the other members of the multidisciplinary mental health team. It is here in the neighborhood around the agency that the community laboratory exists as the proper source of data and as the sounding board for action research. It is here, in short, where the acid test of self-worth as a community mental health research worker is given and scored and where the report card is issued.

The novice researcher must adjust to many problems, and he needs all the sense of trust his earlier training at the university has built into his role repertoire. He discovers quickly that he is not the central actor in the agency drama, that his colleagues are busy with incredibly heavy day-to-day workloads of service, that his administrators are preoccupied politically with winning program acceptance, that the community purse-holders are apt to regard research out of hand as mere frills, and that, on the surface at least, everyone accepts the worth of present services as face-valid and not requiring evaluative research.

Adaptation to this situation, interestingly enough, requires that the researcher use the practitioner skills acquired from earlier community practicum experiences to demonstrate that he feels competent to function as a researcher in such a way as to be of value to the agency and to the community. As Brooks (1965) states, the researcher can provide sensible ideas for experimenting with modifications in agency practice, collect and analyze demographic and other types of data necessary for agency planning, and assist in the planning process itself by helping the staff follow the steps in standard decision-making models. This type of cooperative behavior on the researcher's part is likely to lead automatically to agency sanction and encouragement to design and implement the basic research and program evaluative research that he is committed to as nuclear to his self-image. By way of contrast, if the researcher had come to the field agency without previously achieving a sense of trust and feeling of competence, he would almost certainly fail in turn to achieve an acceptable sense of identity.

REFERENCES

Berne, E. *Games people play.* New York: Grove Press, 1964.

Brooks, M. P. The community action program as a setting for applied research. *J. soc. Issues,* 1965, **21**, 29-40.

Chein, I. Some sources of divisiveness among psychologists. *Amer. Psychologist,* 1966, **21**, 333-342.

Dunnette, M. D. Fads, fashions, and folderol in psychology. *Amer. Psychologist,* 1966, **21**, 343-352.

Gelfand, S., & Kelly, J. G. The psychologist in community mental health: scientist and professional. *Amer. Psychologist,* 1960, **15**, 223-226.

CHAPTER 18

Multiple Functions for Psychologists in Community Consultation[1]

Lester M. Libo

Psychologists are assuming a wider range of responsibilities in community program administration and community consultation: in mental health, corrections, education, and antipoverty. In mental health, for example, they are working as Federal and regional consultants for the National Institute of Mental Health, as state directors and consultants in mental health programs, as mental health planners, as directors and staff members of mental health centers, and as locally based community consultants. University training programs are beginning to place greater emphasis on the potential role of their students in community mental health services. Psychologists have undertaken and completed courses of study in schools of public health. Some have become prominent leaders in the development of new concepts and techniques in public health–mental health programing.

In these roles, psychologists are being asked to deal with many topics which have not traditionally been given much emphasis in

[1]Paper read in "Psychology and Community Mental Health: Prospects and Preparation," symposium presented at American Psychological Association, Chicago, September 1965.

Since this paper was addressed to an audience of psychologists, it necessarily focuses on the role and training of psychologists, with the full realization that psychologists are only one segment of professional services in community mental health. The experiences and recommendations should be applicable to the other mental health disciplines as well.

doctoral training programs, such as alcoholism, narcotics addiction, welfare dependency, unwed mothers, school dropouts, juvenile delinquency, aftercare services for mental patients, the training of volunteers, the preparation of public information materials (in *non*psychological language), the organization of treatment environments, the education of disadvantaged children, the epidemiology of personal and social problems, and comprehensive planning for coordinated community-wide services.

In many states, psychologists, as well as representatives of other disciplines (such as social work, psychiatry, nursing, and education), are functioning as "generalists"—as general practitioners in human welfare services—and, in the smaller communities, are sometimes the only available source of professional expertise, both for developing community resources and for rendering direct services to individuals and groups. Particularly when the psychologist finds himself in the position of being the only mental health consultant in a community, he is faced vividly, dramatically, and often anxiously with the question of how well his academic training, internship, and professional experience have prepared him.

Consultation is being given to practitioners in fields not usually related to the clinical psychologist's traditional practicum experience, such as: lawyers, judges, civic officials, police officers, public welfare workers, teachers, and public health physicians and nurses. Long-term psychotherapy (especially psychoanalysis), Rorschach reports, lengthy intake procedures, close supervision, frequent case conferences, full clinical teams of co-professionals, and other familiar trappings of our typical training environments are often unheard of in the majority of communities—communities which by reason of their overwhelming numbers (and I include, along with rural and small town areas, most neighborhoods in urban areas) represent the mainstream of American life. Nevertheless, to the traditional professional mental health specialist at least, these communities are considered "underdeveloped areas" and, quite mistakenly, atypical or beyond our immediate concern.

Try to envision the demands placed upon your personal and professional skills if you were hired to function as a truly "compleat psychologist," as a representative, say, of a state mental health program, to go into a community as its first and only professional mental health worker, to live there for several years as its "Mr. Mental Health," and to do all you could to develop a locally based program of community services. You would try to serve preventive, therapeutic, and rehabilitative goals, with a full realization that innovative approaches would be necessary, since you, as the lone mental health resource, could not realistically function solely as a clinician dealing with individual cases. You could not conceivably begin to handle the "caseload" yourself. If you tried to do so, if for no other reason than that is what you know and can do most comfortably, you would soon realize that a community program was not being developed, that other resources were not being mobilized, and that trying to stem the tide without paying attention to prevention and collaborative participation by others would soon lead to feelings of desperation and despair.

Instead, if you took your title of "consultant" seriously, your caseload would have to be the entire community's network of agencies, organizations, and practitioners who would turn to you (if you were receptive, supportive, and helpful) with the psychological and social problems in *their* caseloads, with their own need for more knowledge and skill in handling their clients, and with their interest in developing more and better services in the community. Thus, your caseload would consist of *consultees*. Their work with cases and in general community improvement, with your help, would serve the goals of the mental health program. Individuals and families would continue to be helped, it is hoped in improved ways, but more indirectly than directly as far as your own work was concerned; their "treatment" would come largely from "community care givers." The results, it is hoped, would be "therapeutic," though the procedures used would not necessarily be psychotherapy.

It was just such an approach which we developed in New Mexico: the District Mental Health Consultant program. This was a 4-year demonstration project, supported by a National Institute of Mental Health Title V Mental Health Project Grant,[2] beginning in 1959. The approach was analogous to the "county extension agent" format in agriculture, and was designed to start consultation, training, demonstration, and community development activities in four areas of the state that virtually lacked any professional mental health services. For two of these four areas we chose psy-

[2]MH 286: "Mental Health Consultation in Underdeveloped Areas." This project was an integral part of the State mental health program. The writer was Director, Division of Mental Health, New Mexico Department of Public Health, 1957-62.

chologists as our district consultants. In the third area, we assigned a psychiatric social worker, and in the fourth, a nurse–mental health consultant. A psychiatrist with his own airplane was our state-level consultant who, by flying to the districts, which were in the more outlying parts of the state, served the program on a part-time basis to supplement the work of the full-time locally based person, as a medical consultant as well as a general source of support.

The District Mental Health Consultant's office was in the county health department but he was offered to the entire community as "someone to turn to" in helping develop a mental health program befitting its needs and resources. Toward this goal, the consultant's work consisted of four types of activities: (*a*) community organization (including interagency program planning, coordination, and resource development); (*b*) case consultation to agencies and practitioners; (*c*) in-service training to agencies and organizations; (*d*) public information and education. Direct clinical services were also included, but only as a vehicle for accomplishing the other goals—i.e., as a demonstration in consultation, training, and community organization.

The work involved sustained contacts with agencies, organizations, and practitioners in public health, welfare, education, clergy, medicine, recreation, county and municipal government, probation and parole, police departments, courts, hospitals, home extension clubs, civic organizations, and others. There were many varied activities and much travel. The consultant was available as the public mental health professional resource in his district and was open to every conceivable kind of request, as well as having to keep constantly in mind the goals of community organization for mental health.

Districts ranged in size from 2½ to 4 counties. Each district encompassed from three to five major communities of from 10,000 to 35,000 population. Travel distances ranged from about 20 miles to 125 miles between the three to five main stops the consultant made each day or two. In all of the districts, hundreds of miles of travel were required for visiting the major communities. Overnight stays were usually necessary for traveling the full circuit each week. Nevertheless, living in his district placed the consultant much closer to his population than if a state-level traveling team were to be used.

To study and evaluate the development of this program and its impact on the 13 counties in which it was introduced, as well as its impact on the consultants themselves, we employed social science personnel from cultural anthropology, sociology, and social psychology. A careful documentation of all consultation contacts was made by means of daily logs submitted by the consultants, and a coding scheme classified the entries. These revealed that the major kinds of functions performed by the consultants were:

—Getting acquainted and establishing rapport

—Becoming visible as a resource person

—Expediting interagency communication, referrals, and coordination of services

—Providing case consultation services

—Providing direct clinical services (as demonstrations of what they were and could do and for rapport building with strategic agencies and practitioners)

—Conducting mental health education and training programs for professional and lay groups

—Helping to organize and expand mental health or mental health-related facilities

Other activities, but of lesser frequency, were:

—Conducting mental health information programs

—Providing administrative, organizational, and program consultation services to agencies

—Participating in administrative and research procedures, including program evaluation

In looking at this list of activities, as well as the long list of allied professionals contacted and the wide range of topics and projects in which the consultants were involved, we see that some of the consultant's work involves professional psychological skills—in the sense that the work requires concepts and techniques in clinical psychology, social psychology, child development, learning, motivation, etc. Most—or even all—of the knowledge and skill required for the consultant's typical functions, however, are also claimed (and offered) by social work, psychiatry, nursing, and public health–mental health. This is true particularly in counseling with troubled or troublesome people and their care givers, evaluating problem behavior, suggesting courses of action and solutions, making referrals, designing community self-surveys, interviewing for data collection, presenting and interpreting knowledge about mental health content and skills to lay and professional people in the community (such as in a workshop for clergymen, police, or teachers), planning and describing programs for prevention, treatment, and rehabilitation, and helping to organize facilities to carry out such programs.

In many contacts, being a professional and a doctor carries a great deal of status and provides a more convenient entry for the consultant than if he were simply a "mister" or a layman, though this advantage is short-lived and is soon overshadowed by personal attributes and skills. Many of the consultant's major activities, such as "getting acquainted," "establishing rapport," "becoming visible as a resource person," and "expediting interagency communication," are not unique to mental health services. They require skill, not in professional psychology, but in community organization and community development. Yet it is debatable whether they are less difficult, or less important, or less "technical" skills than other professional functions. Because of the constant interaction in community work between knowledge and practice, it is debatable whether the consultant's knowledge is really more fundamentally "psychological" than the techniques he uses to implement it. (This is, after all, a major concern of social psychology, the Society for the Psychological Study of Social Issues, and action research.) It is deceptively easy to dismiss these community activities as "public relations" and to assume that any layman or volunteer could do them, leaving the professional to devote all of his time to specialized, technical work. To the contrary, we found that unless the mental health professional could carefully groom others to help him with some of his community activities, he was the only one equipped to represent his knowledge and skill in getting them implemented in community action. Mental health program development requires frequent and sustained contact between the consultant, his consultees, and their colleagues in the community.

SELECTION OF COMMUNITY CONSULTANTS

The first step in preparing psychologists for broad responsibility in community action is to select the right psychologist for the job. In selecting our district consultants, we used these criteria: (*a*) sound graduate training, including the terminal degree for the profession (PhD for psychologists, master's for social workers and nurses); (b) substantial clinical skills in diagnosis and therapy; (c) experience in consultation and administration; (d) experience in community work. Our experience requirement was 5 years beyond the graduate degree.

These high standards were necessary because the consultant was to be the first and only professional resource person in his district. Independent and responsible action was to be demanded of him constantly.

Personal and social attributes and communication skills are also very important considerations for community consultation work: an outgoing and friendly manner, ability to speak and write clearly and in popular language, humanitarian values, high energy level, broad interests, ability to organize complex material and crystallize it into its essentials, persistence in pursuing long-range goals while being able to tolerate slow progress and short-term setbacks, and, probably most important of all, an abiding dedication and loyalty to program philosophy coupled with a patient, accepting attitude toward the people with whom one works in the community. These attributes should involve an equalitarian and respectful attitude toward people of all social classes, political affiliations, and educational levels. The well-known motto for this is: Start with people where they are. To do this, one must really enjoy frequent and intense interaction with all kinds of people, especially nonprofessionals, and to be able to forgo the cautious, perfectionistic, intellectualized, and even condescending manner sometimes seen in professionals. Some traits that academicians value are often associated in the public mind with deviousness and dishonesty, not to mention inadequacy, inefficiency, and weakness. You do not answer a question with a question, and you do not hedge everything you say until no one knows what you have really said. Particularly in smaller communities, a straightforward, open, and robust mode of communication and social interaction are favored. Condescension ("airs") and jargon ("gobbledygook") are anathema.

ORIENTATION

After we selected and hired our consultants, we conducted a 2-month, full-time orientation program for them—this involved a great deal of reading on various mental health topics, techniques, and programs; discussions and readings on state and local geography, history, economics, culture, politics, and health, education, and welfare services; visits to all relevant state agencies and institutions with which the consultant would be working after moving to his district; interviews with state government officials, university faculty members, and others who knew local conditions and personalities, including the state chairmen of the Democratic and Republican parties; and reviews of all state office files and correspondence pertaining to interests, needs, and resources in the local district.

All four consultants valued the orientation program greatly. None felt really prepared for the role of a lone consultant. None had been in such a role before. When comparing one mental health profession to another, we found that none really prepared its people for such a role. We base this conclusion on the opinions of the professions themselves (when they let their hair down), on the feelings of the district consultants we hired, and on our recruitment experience which involved the applications of 57 psychologists and 11 social workers. (We hired the first nurse and the first psychiatrist we contacted, so lengthy recruitment was not necessary for those two professions.) Of the social workers and psychologists, too many, unfortunately, had no conception of prevention, consultation, community organization, or interagency coordination. They were familiar and comfortable only with diagnosis and/or treatment in a highly structured setting. Such "conservatism" was particularly strong among women.

Those we selected were different. In some ways they were mavericks. They were dissatisfied with traditional modes of clinical practice, they wanted more personal and professional autonomy, and they felt strong enough to stand alone as a community resource. They were, needless to say, adventurous.

Nevertheless, they needed and wanted more preparation. The orientation program helped them, all agreed, but when the consultants finally moved to their respective districts, their automobiles loaded with dictating machines, pamphlets, brochures, reference materials, and names of potentially helpful contacts, they, in all cases, showed a mixture of eagerness and panic.[3]

---

[3]The State office staff had done some preparatory work with community groups and agencies in the four districts prior to the consultants' arrival, but the consult-

Within the first few weeks of their new life in their districts, and for the duration of their work there (which ranged from 1 year to 5 years), they experienced the gamut of reactions from triumph to despair. Though there were varying levels of success, from extremely high to minimal, all four, nevertheless, made positive contributions.

ACCOMPLISHMENTS

The New Mexico mental health consultation project stimulated the development of the following new resources in local communities:

—A day school for retarded children
—A mental health *checkup* project for second-grade children
—A family casework agency
—A day center for emotionally disturbed children
—A training and consultation service to an orphanage
—Training and consultation services to school teachers, law enforcement workers, and clergymen
—The selection and training of nonprofessional community project leaders and volunteers for work in a comprehensive local mental health program
—An alcoholism treatment and rehabilitation program for Navajo Indians
—Formation of citizens' organizations for planning and supporting local mental health services
—Formation of parents' organizations for retarded and emotionally disturbed children
—Organization of *case panels* to assemble all relevant expertise around an individual or family mental health problem, for planning and coordinating a unified program of early detection and community management, using existing local resources

These services were developed over the 4-year project period, and virtually all of them, as well as many new ones, have continued in operation to this day. It is worthy of note that almost all local services in the 13 New Mexico communities included in the project districts were developed only after professional mental health consultants were made available to these communities as locally based fellow citizens. Before the establishment of the project, a ants did not find these contacts to be sufficient either in number or in motivation to support a substantial community organization effort.

decade of experimentation with traveling teams and periodic "clinics" conducted by nonresidents had resulted in no local mental health services that could be sustained.

TOURISM IS NOT ENOUGH*

Many psychologists spend their careers working in the houses of other professions—medicine, psychiatry, public health, industrial management, and education. In these settings, psychologists and other behavioral scientists are sometimes accused of being aloof and peripheral, "permanent, floating consultants," always ready to offer the complacent wisdom of uncommitted, detached observers who do not man the night shift or the emergency room. We will often discuss the philosophical or theoretical implications of the others' programs, point to shortcomings of their models, suggest promising and creative new approaches, and constantly embarrass by asking about evaluation of effectiveness. At the same time, we lecture about the multivariate roots of human behavior, the importance of sociocultural context, and the unity of man and his environment. Yet, we tend neither to immerse ourselves in those very environments of human existence and human problem solving with which the civic officials, educators, physicians, police officers, public-health nurses, and welfare workers deal so closely and painfully each day, nor to assume the responsibilities of command (the only way we can really influence the system). We are often commentators in other men's arenas, visiting professors in other men's schools.

When we work in psychology's own houses—such as in a psychological research institute or a psychological service center—we tend to give up the role of critical observer and become more committed to the goals of the organization and indeed we do man the night shifts and respond to emergency calls. Often in programs that are under psychologists' auspices, it will be the other professionals—psychiatrists, sociologists, educators, mathematicians— who are in "staff" rather than in "line" roles, and *they* are the peripheral ones, the technical consultants, the commentators on *our* scene. They see the big holes in our line, and, I am sure, they are sometimes disdained and even resented by those in charge.

*This section (original publication in this book) is based on the author's presentation at the symposium, "Issues and Trends in Community Psychology Training," 74th Annual Convention of the American Psychological Association, New York City, September 2, 1966.

We should be concerned about the role models we will offer our new generation of community-psychology trainees. Community psychology should not be another haven for marginal man or another perch from which to snipe at those in charge. When community psychologists are trained, they must be trained by immersion in, not only exposure to, community life. The visiting professor, particularly if he is a gadfly, is not an adequate role model—at least not for a young apprentice. Nor is the trainee-tourist, who samples an hour in one agency, a day in another, a week in another, and goes back to the comfortable rear-echelon, knowing that he will not need to commit himself, his theories, and his methodologies to the test of policy and practice for which he himself will be held responsible.

An apprenticeship in community psychology must involve the assumption of sustained, responsible roles in community work—in appraisal of community characteristics and in performance of community-management tasks. Psychologists must get the experience of managing community institutions and community programs. Psychologists have many areas of expertise to bring to bear on community needs—child development, learning, motivation, group process, attitude and opinion measurement, personality assessment, behavior modification. Conversely, community structure and dynamics, and the wide variety of social problems in communities, have much to offer scientific psychology (by providing a natural laboratory for observing and modifying behavior), as well as professional psychological practice (by providing the challenge of solving problems in their natural environments). In fact, community psychology might well be an organizing focus for all of applied psychology, since it does seem to call upon all psychological subspecialties, as varied as social psychology, consumer psychology, engineering psychology, clinical psychology, educational psychology, child psychology, and experimental physiological psychology. (The last-mentioned field is often associated with "pure" research and with the "scientist" side of the lamentable scientist-practitioner schism in psychology today, but it should be remembered that psychopharmacology and bio-astronautics are both "applied" fields that are eminently respectable consumers of the consulting services of psychological scientists. The same trend is becoming evident with regard to learning theorists and behavior therapy.)

The delightful thing about psychology is that it encompasses every aspect of behavior and therefore allows the imaginative and creative psychologist to direct his professional concern to almost any human problem. Many psychologists have shed their detached, peripheral roles regarding human and social improvement and have conducted community programs of major significance. Sometimes they are asked if there is anything distinctively psychological about what they are doing or whether they, by becoming activists, have blurred their identities and become generic "mental-healthers" or "community-development specialists," indistinguishable from their counterparts in other disciplines.

We need not be worried about the effect of this question either on the community psychologist or on society. He is identifiable by his function more than by his discipline presumably because society values the doing of real jobs more than it does the identification of professional territoriality. His academic ancestry will be appreciated when it contributes to his success in community programs.

If the university, in partnership with community institutions, agencies, and practitioners, can become a force for integrating all of "a compleat psychology," and provide training formats and role models which demonstrate this partnership in action, the professor, the researcher, and the practitioner will benefit. What is even more important, their students and trainees will no longer have to be tourists in their own land.

Index of Names

Index of Topics

7